MANUAL OF CLINICAL BLOOD TRANSFUSION

Branko Brozovic PhD, MRCPath
Consultant Haematologist,
North London Blood Transfusion
Centre & Regional Blood Transfusion Service,
London, UK

Milica Brozovic FRCPath
Consultant Haematologist,
Central Middlesex Hospital,
London, UK

Churchill Livingstone

EDINBURGH LONDON MELBOURNE AND NEW YORK 1986

CHURCHILL LIVINGSTONE
Medical Division of Longman Group Limited

Distributed in the United States of America by Churchill Livingstone Inc., 1560 Broadway, New York, N.Y. 10036, and by associated companies, branches and representatives throughout the world.

First published 1986

ISBN 0-443-02874-5

British Library Cataloguing in Publication Data
Brozovic, Branko
    Manual of clinical blood transfusion. — (Manuals series)
    1. Blood — Transfusion
    I. Title   II. Brozovic, Milica
    615'.65   RM171

Library of Congress Cataloging in Publication Data
Brozovic, Branko
    Manual of clinical blood transfusion.
    (Manuals series)
    Includes index.
    1. Blood — Transfusion — Handbooks, manuals, etc.
I. Brozovic, Milica.   II. Title. [DNLM: 1. Blood Transfusion — handbooks.
WB 39 B885m]
RM171.B75   1985   615'.65   85-11710

Produced by Longman Singapore, Publishers (Pte) Ltd.
Printed in Singapore.

MANUAL OF CLINICAL
BLOOD TRANSFUSION

Already published

Paediatric Gastroenterology *J.H. Tripp and D.C.A. Candy*
Renal Disease *C.B. Brown*
Haematology *A.S.J. Baughan, A.S.B. Hughes, K.G. Patterson and L. Stirling*
Chest Medicine *J.E. Stark, J.M. Shneerson, T. Higenbottam and C.D.R. Flower*

Forthcoming volumes in the Manuals series

Gastroenterology *B.T. Cooper and R.E. Barry*
Cardiology *K. Dawkins*
Infectious Diseases *J.A. Innes*
Rheumatology *J.M.H. Moll*
Neonatal Intensive Care *A.R. Wilkinson*
Gynaecology *T.R. Varma*

PREFACE

The purpose of this manual is to describe the clinical practice of blood transfusion with particular emphasis on the management of patients and the rational use of blood, blood components and products. The manual is intended for junior medical staff requesting and administering blood transfusions on the ward or in the operating theatre. We hope, however, that medical, technical and scientific staff involved with blood transfusions in haematological departments, blood banks and blood transfusion centres, as well as medical students and nurses, will find the manual informative.

We would like to thank Professor G.I.C. Ingram for reading the manuscript and for his, always constructive, comments. Many colleagues have given us generous advice on technical and theoretical problems and we would like to thank them all, in particular Dr J.A.J. Barbara, Mr J.G. Bennett, Dr Sally Davies, Mr A. Devenish, Mrs Margot Gibson, Mr G. Hazelhurst, Miss Joan Henthorn, Mr R. Knight, Dr Elizabeth Letsky, Mr J. Martin, Mr A McWilliam, Dr Valerie Mijović, Dr C.V. Petersen, Dr Gizelle Schwarz and Dr V. Šljivić. For the shortcomings of the manual we alone are responsible.

We are indebted to Mrs Margaret Geary for her skill and patience in typing the manuscript, Mrs Irene Prentice for the excellent illustrations and Mr M. Etherington for photographic work.

London, 1986

B.B.
M.B.

CONTENTS

1. RED CELL SYSTEMS OF ANTIGENS AND CORRESPONDING ANTIBODIES

ANTIGENS, ANTIBODIES AND ANTIGEN-ANTIBODY REACTION

There are many *antigens* on the surface of red cells, white cells and platelets. Each are capable of stimulating the production of a corresponding *antibody* when administered to a person who lacks them. A few of these antigens are shared by cells of different types. For example, the antigens of the ABO and HLA systems are present on almost all cells in the body, although their expression may vary in strength. The majority of other antigens, however, are found only on one type of cell, e.g. red cells, granulocytes, lymphocytes or platelets. In addition, some plasma proteins possess antigenic determinants which may stimulate the production of alloantibodies following transfusion to a recipient who lacks them.

The immune response normally follows the encounter with an alloantigen, that is an antigen which is recognised as 'foreign' by the immune recognition system. The immune response is the end result of interaction between the antigen, macrophages, T lymphocytes and B lymphocytes. After activation B lymphocytes are transformed into secretory plasma cells and produce the specific antibody. The antibodies produced in the *primary response*, when the alloantigen is introduced into the organism for the first time, are IgM immunoglobulins. A proportion of antibodies produced at a later stage of the primary response may be IgG immunoglobulins. A *secondary response* (anamnestic response) is brought about by a second or subsequent encounter(s) with the same alloantigen. In the secondary response the rate of antibody production is faster and the concentration of antibody much higher than in the primary response. The antibodies produced are predominantly IgG immunoglobulins. On rare occasions, some of the antibodies produced may be IgA immunoglobulins.

An *antigen-antibody reaction* involving red cells leads to their agglutination or destruction; the many factors governing those processes are described in detail in Chapter 9. Only reactions which result in shortening the lifespan of red cells are of clinical importance. Red cell lifespan is reduced either by predominantly intravascular direct lysis by complement binding (haemolytic) antibodies such as anti-A and anti-B, or by destruction of red cells sequestered in the spleen, brought about by antibodies which do not bind complement (non-haemolytic), such as the anti-K. Similarly, antibodies to platelets or granulocytes can shorten the lifespan of these cells.

Red cell antigens and the corresponding antibodies are described in this chapter, the platelet and leucocyte antigens and their corresponding antibodies, and plasma protein antigens and their corresponding antibodies in Chapter 4.

Red cell antigens

Red cell antigens are substances on the surface of the red cell which can stimulate the formation of antibodies. There are over 400 antigens recognised, but each person possesses only a small proportion of that number. Red cell antigens are grouped into many systems, but only a few are of clinical importance; this depends almost entirely on (i) the ability of the antibodies in the system to destroy red cells in vivo, and (ii) the frequency of occurrence of antibodies in a population.

The *molecular structure* which determines antigenic specificity has been worked out for only a small number of red cell antigens. For example, the antigenic specificity of A, B and H antigens is determined by the type and site of attachment of the terminal sugars, that of M, N, S and s antigens depends on a combination of the amino acid sequence and sugar structure of the molecule; and that of Rh antigens is governed by the amino acid sequence in the presence of specific phospholipids.

Genes carried on autosomal chromosomes determine the molecular structure of antigens. Some red cell antigens, such as Rh and K antigens which are proteins, are direct gene products. Others, such as A, B, H, Le^a and Le^b antigens, are the end result of the action of the gene product, which is a specific enzyme. This transfers a sugar molecule onto a protein or lipid backbone, whose structure is in turn determined by another, unrelated, gene.

The *inheritance* of blood groups follows the Mendelian pattern. Genes which may occupy the same locus on a pair of homologous chromosomes are called *allelic genes* or *alleles*. When both loci are occupied by the same genes the person is *homozygous*, or when two different but allelic genes occupy the same loci the person is *heterozygous*, for that particular blood group. For the only blood group carried on the X chromosome, Xg^a, a woman can be homo- or heterozygous, whereas a man can only be hemizygous having only one X chromosome (Fig. 1.1).

The *genotype* of a given characteristic denotes all the inherited genes which code for it, and the *phenotype* denotes the recognisable features of that characteristic in an individual. However, some genes produce no recognisable effect on any chemical structure. Such genes are called *amorphic genes* or *amorphs*. For example, homozygosity for two

(A)

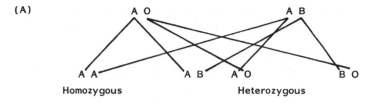

(B)

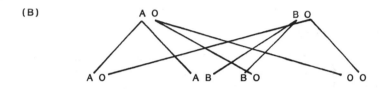

(C)

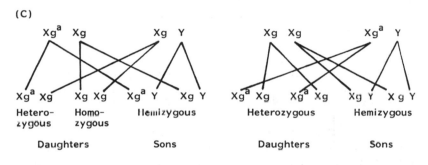

Fig. 1.1 Inheritance of genes determining the red cell antigens: (A) Inheritance of the ABO genes, homozygous and heterozygous individuals. (B) Offspring of parents with genotype AO and BO can have phenotypes A, AB, B and O. (C) Inheritance of X-linked Xgᵃ and Xg genes. When the mother carries the Xgᵃ gene, daughters can be heterozygous or homozygous for Xg while the sons are hemizygous. When the father carries the Xgᵃ gene the daughters are heterozygous and the sons hemizygous.

amorphic genes O, and the absence of the end product, determines the specificity of blood group O. The presence of an amorphic gene in a heterozygote can be deduced only by a family study.

Frequencies of genes, genotypes and phenotypes Gene frequency represents the fraction of the population who possess the specified gene. For example, the gene frequencies for Jk^a and Jk^b are 0.514 and 0.486, respectively. There are three genotypes, Jk^aJk^a, Jk^aJk^b and Jk^bJk^b, and their frequencies, expressed as a percentage, are calculated as follows: for Jk^aJk^a, $0.514 \times 0.514 \times 100 = 25.9\%$; for Jk^bJk^b, $0.486 \times 0.486 \times 100 = 23.6\%$, for Jk^aJk^b, $0.514 \times 0.486 \times 2 \times 100 = 49.9\%$; multiplication by 2 is required to account for the fact that Jk^a can combine with Jk^b, but also that Jk^b can combine with Jk^b. The frequencies of phenotypes Jk(a+b−),

Jk(a+b+) and Jk(a−b+)are the same as that of genotypes Jk^aJk^a, Jk^aJk^b and Jk^bJk^b, also expressed as a percentage. However, the frequency of antigen Jk^a,that is to say the phenotype Jk(a+), is 75.8% and that of antigen Jk^b, the phenotype Jk(b+), is 73.5%. When using gene frequencies the population investigated should be precisely specified, because gene frequencies may vary considerably in different ethnic groups.

Antibodies to red cell antigens

Antibodies are immunoglobulins which react specifically with corresponding antigens. There are five classes of immunoglobulins: IgM, IgG, IgA, IgD and IgE, of which only the first two are important in blood transfusion. Red cell antibodies of the IgA class appear rarely and then almost invariably together with IgM and IgG antibodies. The main properties of IgG, IgM and IgA immunoglobulins are shown in Table 1.1.

Table 1.1 Main properties of IgG, IgM, and IgA immunoglobulins

Property	Class of immunoglobulin		
	IgG	IgM	IgA
Structure	monomer	pentamer	monomer
Molecular weight, daltons	150 000	900 000	150 000
Sedimentation constant	75	195	75
Concentration in plasma, g/l	6–16	0.5–1.5	1.5–4.5
Extravascular pool, % of total body content	56	20	60
Antigen binding sites per molecule	2	5 or 10	2
Complement fixation	occasionally	usually and efficiently	none
Transfer across placenta	yes	no	no

Antibodies are produced in response to immunisation by an antigen. *Autoantibodies* are antibodies that react with antigens present on the person's own red cells, and sometimes, in autoimmune diseases, with antigens present on the red cells of other normal individuals (see also Ch. 9). *Alloantibodies* are antibodies produced by the person against antigens (alloantigens) lacking on the person's own red cells. Alloantibodies can be naturally occurring or immune (i.e. induced by contact with the antigen).

Naturally occurring red cell antibodies are found in a person who has never received blood or blood products, or vaccines of human origin, has never been pregnant nor undergone organ transplantation, and may arise through one of two mechanisms. First, it seems possible that some immunocompetent cells may be capable of producing a specific antibody in the absence of an antigenic stimulus. Second, the antibodies may be produced in response to substances present in the environment and antigenically similar to blood group antigens.

Immune antibodies arise as a result of exposure to an alloantigen by transfusion of blood or blood products, pregnancy, vaccination with vaccines of human origin, or transplantation. The production of immune antibodies mainly depends on:

1. The properties of the alloantigen. Some blood group antigens, such as D, are more immunogenic than the others. Other potent immunogens are K, c, Fy^a and Jk^a.
2. The dose of antigen and mode of exposure. The risk of producing immune antibodies increases with administration of large, repeated and frequent doses of antigen. Transfusion carries a higher risk of inducing immunisation than pregnancy.
3. The individual response of the recipient. Some individuals are 'good responders' and promptly produce immune antibodies in a high titre, whereas others rarely if ever produce antibodies, even after repeated attempts to immunise them. The main properties of naturally occurring and immune antibodies are shown in Table 1.2.

Table 1.2 Main characteristics of naturally occurring and immune antibodies to red cell antigens

Characteristic	Naturally occurring antibodies	Immune antibodies
Immunoglobulin class	IgM	IgM early in primary response, IgG late in primary response and in secondary response
Complement fixation	usually and efficiently	occasionally
Optimal temperature for agglutination	cold, rarely reactive at temperatures higher than 25°C	warm, rarely reactive at temperatures lower than 30°C
In vitro behaviour	complete antibody (agglutinating in saline), haemolytic	incomplete antibody (coating red cells), occasionally agglutinating in saline and haemolytic
Clinical significance	mostly harmless, but haemolytic transfusion reaction for antibodies of the ABO system	haemolytic transfusion reaction and haemolytic disease of the newborn
Blood group systems against which the antibodies are usually found	ABO, Lewis, P, Ii*	Rhesus, Kell, Duffy, (ABO)

* Naturally occurring antibodies in other blood group systems have been described but they are very rare.

Blood group terminology

Blood group systems are represented by the full name of the system or denoted by an abbreviation. For example, the ABO, Kell and Duffy systems are denoted as ABO, K and Fy systems.

Genes are denoted by capital letters in italics with superscript where appropriate. In some systems allelic genes are denoted both by capital and small letters. For example, genes *H* and *A¹* in the ABO system, allelic genes *Se* and *se* which determine the secretory status, and genes *Le^a* and *Le^b* in the Lewis system.

Antigens are denoted by capital and small letters with appropriate subscripts or superscripts. For example, antigens M,N,S and s in the MNSs system, antigens A_1 and A_2 in the ABO system and antigens Lu^a and Lu^b in the Lutheran system.

Phenotypes are presented to indicate presence or absence of a given antigen. For example, Fy(a+b−) shows that Fy^a was detected on the red cells but Fy^b was not detected.

Antibodies are written as follows: anti-A_1, anti-K, anti-Fy^a. The presence of two antibodies in the same serum sample is denoted as follows: anti-C+D.

The terminology used for the Rh system follows in principle that used for other blood groups. However, different nomenclatures are used for antigens of the Rh system, and these will be described later.

THE ABO SYSTEM

This is the first system of red cell antigens described and also the most important one, because naturally occurring antibodies, found in all individuals who do not possess the corresponding antigen(s), are capable of producing a rapid and complete intravascular haemolysis of incompatible red cells. The ensuing haemolytic transfusion reaction is often serious and occasionally fatal.

Antigens of the ABO system

Genes, gene products and gene frequencies

Three allelic genes, *A*, *B* and *O*, and a pair of allelic genes, *H* and *h*, are responsible for the formation of antigens A and B (Table 1.3). Gene *H* codes for enzyme H (α-L-fucosyltransferase) which attaches a molecule of fucose to the glycoprotein backbone of the precursor substance to form substance H. Gene *h* is an amorphic gene without an end product. Genes *A* and *B* code for enzyme A (α-N-acetyl-D-galactosaminyl-transferase) and

Table 1.3 The ABO system, genes, gene frequencies, gene products and antigens*

Gene	Gene frequency*	Gene product (enzyme)	Molecule attached	Antigen (serological specificity)
H	very high	α-L-fucosyltransferase	fucose	H
h	very low	none	—	—
A	0.2573	α-N-acetyl-D-galactosaminyltransferase (enzyme A)	galactos-amine	A
B	0.0600	α-D-galactosyltransferase (enzyme B)	galactose	B
O	0.6827	none	—	—

* In Britain

enzyme B (α-D-galactosyltransferase), respectively. Enzyme A attaches a molecule of galactosamine, and enzyme B a molecule of galactose, to substance H, and thus provide antigenic specificity for antigens A and B. Gene O is an amorph without an end product. The gene frequencies in Britain are shown in Table 1.4.

Table 1.4 The ABO system. Genotypes, phenotypes, antibodies in serum and the incidence of blood groups*

Genotype	Agglutination by antibodies	Antibodies in the serum	Blood group	Incidence, %
A^1A^1, A^1O**	anti-A+A$_1$	anti-B	A$_1$	35 ⎫ 45
A^2A^2, A^2O	anti-A	anti-B†	A$_2$	10 ⎭
BB, BO	anti-B	anti-A	B	8
A^1B	anti-A+A$_1$+B	none	A$_1$B	2.5 ⎫ 3
A^2B	anti-A+B	none‡	A$_2$B	0.5 ⎭
OO	none	anti-A+A$_1$+B	O	44

* In Britain
** Persons of the genotype A^1A^2 cannot be detected by serological testing, but they possess A^1 and A^2 transferases in the serum which differ qualitatively and quantitatively, although both transferases have the same specificity.
† 2% of persons possess an anti-A$_1$ antibody in the serum.
‡ 25% of persons possess an anti-A$_1$ antibody in the serum.

Genotypes, phenotypes and subgroups of A and B
Genotypes, phenotypes and the incidence of blood groups within the ABO system are shown in Table 1.4.

Subgroups A$_1$ and A$_2$
Two subgroups, A$_1$ and A$_2$, are recognised on group A red cells, using serological reactions. Anti-A antibody agglutinates red cells of both subgroups, but only subgroup A$_1$ cells are agglutinated by anti-A$_1$ antibody or the lectin from the seed of the plant *Dolichos biflorus* (Table 1.5). It appears that the difference in agglutinability by anti-A and anti-

Table 1.5 The ABO system. Serological reactions with blood group A$_1$ and A$_2$

Specificity of antibody	Blood group	
	A$_1$	A$_2$
Anti-A	+	+
Anti-A$_1$	+	—

A$_1$ antibodies is not a qualitative one, but depends on the number of antigen sites, which are reduced on blood group A$_2$ cells. About 1 to 2% of individuals with blood group A$_2$ and some 25% of those with blood group A$_2$B have an anti-A$_1$ antibody, usually naturally occurring.

Other subgroups of A, A$_{int}$, A$_3$, A$_4$, A$_x$, A$_m$, A$_{el}$, and A$_{end}$, have been described. They are all characterised by a reduced number of antigen sites on the surface of the red cells, and consequently by a weak serological reaction with anti-A antibody. The serum often contains anti-A$_1$ antibody. There are other subtle differences between the subgroups of

A. The clinical significance of subgroups of A comes to light only when there is a failure in detecting the A antigen on red cells. When the error is made on the recipient's blood the consequences are rarely serious as compatible, group O red cells are transfused. However, when the error is made on donor cells, blood is incorrectly grouped as O instead of A and the group O recipient, who has anti-A in the plasma, may suffer a serious haemolytic transfusion reaction.

Subgroups of B are much less frequent than the subgroups of A. There is no equivalent to A_2, but B_3, B_x, and B_{el} have been described. They, too, are characterised by a weakened serological reaction with anti-B antibodies.

Expression of A, B and H antigens (substances) in the body fluids
The presence of these antigens in plasma, saliva and seminal fluid depends on the person's secretory status which is under the control of two allelic genes, *Se*, required for the expression of the secretory status, and *se*, an amorphic gene. The genotype of secretors is *SeSe* or *Sese* (homozygous and heterozygous secretors, respectively) and they secrete A, B and H substances in the body fluids depending on their *ABH* genotype. In the individuals with the genotype *sese*, A, B and H are not secreted in the body fluids, although they are fully expressed on the red cells. In Britain 80% of people are secretors.

Effect of disease on the ABO blood group
In leukaemia an apparent weakening of the A antigen in patients with group A, and a similar weakening of antigens B and H have been described. The acquired B antigen has been observed in some A_1 individuals with carcinoma of the colon.

Blood group O_h 'Bombay'
This very rare blood group was first described in a patient from Bombay. Persons with blood group O_h possess genotype *hh* and consequently the substance H is missing from the surface of the red cells. As substance H is the substrate for enzymes A and B, antigens A and B are not expressed whether the genes *A* and *B* are inherited or not. The red cells are not agglutinated by anti-A, anti-B or anti-H antibodies, and an anti-H antibody is present in the serum. A patient whose blood group is O_h can receive only O_h blood.

Antibodies of the ABO system

The *naturally occurring antibodies* are anti-A, anti-A_1, anti-B and anti-H (for details see Table 1.6). They are usually IgM immunoglobulins which bind complement and are sometimes frankly haemolytic in vitro. *Immune antibodies* may be anti-A, anti-A_1, or anti-B. They are usually IgG immunoglobulins, although mixtures with IgM and IgA can be found; many antibodies fix complement and are haemolytic, they invariably react at 37°C and are present in serum in high titre. Both naturally occurring and immune ABO antibodies can cause haemolytic transfusion reaction

Table 1.6 The naturally occurring antibodies of the ABO system

Type of antibody	Blood group	Antibody frequency within the given blood group, %
Anti-A+A$_1$	O	100
	B	100
Anti-B	A$_2$	2
	A$_2$B	25
Anti-A$_1$	O	100
	A	100
Anti-H*	O$_h$	100

* Cold anti-H autoantibody is described on p. 140.

but only the latter cause haemolytic disease of the newborn (Ch. 13).

A *'dangerous universal donor'* is a donor of group O whose serum contains high titre of IgG antibodies, anti-A or anti-B or both, and whose plasma, when administered to a recipient of blood group A, B or AB, can cause haemolysis of the recipient's red cells (see also p. 91).

THE LEWIS SYSTEM*

The main characteristic of the antigens within the Lewis system is that they are soluble substances present in saliva and plasma, which are absorbed from the plasma onto the surface of red cells.

Antigens of the Lewis system

Genes, gene products and gene frequencies
There are two allelic genes, *Le* and *le*. The expression of Le antigen depends on the interaction of *Le* and *le* with genes *H* and *h*, and *Se* and *se*, and it is modified by the ABO phenotype (Table 1.7). The gene product of *Le* is an enzyme, α-L-fucosyltransferase which attaches one molecule of fucose to the precursor substance to give rise to the antigen Le^a, and one molecule of fucose to H substance to give rise to the antigen Le^b. Gene *le* is an amorph.

Genotypes, phenotypes and phenotype frequencies are shown in Table 1.7. At birth Le^a and Le^b are not expressed and all infants are Le(a−b−), by eight weeks of life most infants are Le(a+b−), and at the age of two the Lewis antigens have reached their normal adult pattern. Le(a−b−) phenotype in adults is found in up to 40% of some people of African origin.

* Although the Rh system is next to the ABO system in clinical importance, the Lewis, P and Ii systems are described first, because they all have some of the following features in common: molecular structure, interaction between independently inherited genes, presence of antigens (substances) in saliva and plasma, and a high incidence of naturally occurring antibodies.

Table 1.7 Interaction of genes of the Lewis and secretor status systems; genotypes, phenotypes and phenotype frequencies

Genotype	Lewis substances		Phenotype *	Phenotype frequency,** %
	Present in saliva	Present on red cells		
Le, Se†	Le^a, Le^b	Le^b	Le(b+)	75
Le, sese	Le^a	Le^a	Le(a+)	20
lele, Se	none	none	Le(a−b−)	5

* For subjects of the blood group A_1 and B. Subjects of the blood group A_2 and O with genes *Le, Se* and *H* may have the phenotype Le(a+b+).
** In Britain
† *H* gene is necessary for the formation of Le^b substance.

Antibodies of the Lewis system

Antibodies of the Lewis system are anti-Le^a and anti-Le^b. Naturally occurring antibodies are common, often with a wide thermal range. They are usually harmless, reacting best at room temperature, but several cases of haemolytic transfusion reactions have been described. Immune antibodies are rare and haemolytic disease of the newborn has not been reported, presumably because all infants are Le(a−b−) at birth. For transfusion of recipients with anti-Le^a and anti-Le^b antibodies reacting at 37°C see p. 91.

THE P SYSTEM

Antigens of the P system

Genes, gene products and gene frequencies
The exact relationship between three genes P^k, P and P^1, which take part in two different metabolic pathways, is not clear. Gene P^k codes for an enzyme that converts trihexosyl ceramide into globoside (P antigen). In the rare individuals who lack P gene, only trihexosyl ceramide is found on the red cells. Gene P^1 is independent and codes for a transferase that converts paragloboside into the P_1 antigen. In the absence of genes P^k, P and P^1, the individual is said to have the phenotype p.

Genotypes, phenotypes and phenotype frequencies are shown in Table 1.8.

Antibodies of the P system

Anti-P_1 is a common naturally occurring antibody found in about 60% of P_2 individuals and in about 90% of P_2 pregnant women. It only exceptionally causes in vivo haemolysis. Other antibodies in the same

Table 1.8 The P system. Genotypes, phenotypes, antigens and their frequency

Genes coding for antigens			Phenotype	Antigens on red cells	Antibodies in serum	Phenotype frequency, %
P^k	P	P_1				
P^k	P	P^l	P_1	P, P_1	none	75
P^k	P	—	P_2	P	anti-P_1*	25
P^k	—	P^l	P^k_1	P_1, P^k	anti-P	very rare
P^k	—	—	P^k_2	P^k	anti-P	very rare
—	—	—	p	none	anti-$P+P_1+P^k$ (anti-Tj^a)	very rare

* Not present in all P_2 subjects

system are very rare; they are anti-P in some P_1^k or P_2^k individuals and anti-$P+P_1+p^k$(anti-Tj^a) in p individuals. The Donath-Landsteiner antibody commonly has anti-P specificity and it is described on p. 139.

THE Ii SYSTEM

Antigens of the Ii system

The genetic control of I and i antigens is not clear. Antigens of the Ii system are glycoproteins present on the red cells of all individuals. At birth red cells react strongly with anti-i and weakly with anti-I antibodies. During the first year and a half this is gradually changed to the normal adult reaction, strong with anti-I and weak with anti-i. Many diseases, including aplastic, sideroblastic, haemolytic and megaloblastic anaemias, as well as leukaemias, can modify the expression of Ii antigens and enhance the reactivity with anti-i.

Antibodies of the Ii system

Antibodies of the Ii system are cold agglutinins described on p. 140.

THE RHESUS SYSTEM

The clinical importance of the Rhesus (Rh) system is only second to that of the ABO system, because, first, two thirds of Rh(D) negative individuals become immunised after exposure to Rh(D)positive red cells, and second, the antibodies which develop can cause severe haemolytic transfusion reaction and haemolytic disease of the newborn. A small proportion of individuals may become immunised after exposure to antigens of the Rh system other than D.

The antigens of the Rh system

Genes, gene products and gene frequencies
According to the Fisher-Race theory there are three pairs of allelic genes:
D and *d*, *C* and *c*, *E* and *e*. They occupy three loci on chromosome 1,
are closely linked and are inherited as triplets, each triplet containing one
gene from each pair. Rh antigens are proteins but require red cell
phospholipids for expression; they are direct gene products. The presence
of d antigen has not yet been demonstrated and it is conventionally taken
that the silent gene *d* is present in the triplet in the absence of D antigen.
In addition, some 30 other Rh antigens have been recognised on the red
cells. The notation based on the Fisher-Race theory describes the likely
phenotype as two triplets.

In contrast, the Wiener theory postulates that the entire expression of
the Rh system is controlled by a series of genes each occupying only one
locus on the chromosome. Therefore, the Wiener notation used symbols
for the description of the Rh phenotype. The comparison of the two
notations is presented in Table 1.9.

Table 1.9 The Rhesus system. Common gene complexes and their frequency

Gene complex		Frequency*
Fisher-Race notation	Wiener notation	
CDe	R^1	0.4076
cde	*r*	0.3886
cDE	R^2	0.1411
cDe	R^0	0.0257**
C^wDe	R^{1w}	0.0129
cdE	*r″*	0.0119
Cde	*r′*	0.0098
CDE	R^2	rare
CdE	*r^y*	rare

* In the British population
** Common in Negroes

Genotypes, phenotypes and their frequencies are shown in Table 1.10.

Table 1.10 The Rhesus system. Genotypes, phenotypes and their frequencies*

Phenotype	Most common genotype	Genotype frequency %	Alternative genotype	Genotype frequency, %
CcDee	*CDe/cde* (R^1r)	32.0	*CDe/cDe*(R^1R^0)	2
CCDee	*CDe/CDe* (R^1R^1)	17.0	*CDe/Cde* ($R^1r′$)	0.7
ccDEe	*cDE/cde* (R^2r)	11.0	*cDE/cDe* (R^2R^0)	0.7
ccDEE	*cDE/cDE* (R^2R^2)	2.0	*cDE/cdE* ($R^2r″$)	0.3
CcDEe	*CDe/cDE* (R^1R^2)	12.0	*CDe/cdE* ($R^1r″$)	1.0
			cDE/Cde ($R^2r′$)	0.3
			CDE/cde (R^zr)	0.2
ccDee	*cDe/cde* (R^0r)	2.0	*cDe/cDe* (R^0R^0)	0.07*
ccee	*cde/cde* (*rr*)	15.0	none	
Ccee	*Cde/cde* (*r′r*)	1.0	*Cde/Cde* (*r′r′*)	0.02
cceE	*cdE/cde* (*r″r*)	0.9	*cdE/cdE* (*r″r′*)	0.01

* In Negroes the genotype frequency is much higher.
Data from Race RR and Sanger R (1975)

The term Rh 'positive' is used for a person who possesses the D antigen, and conversely the term Rh 'negative' is used for a person who lacks it. However, in the Western world blood transfusion services samples of blood are fully Rh phenotyped and only those which are cde/cde, that is lack C, D and E antigens, are labelled as Rh 'negative'. That is done to extend the protection of the Rh-negative recipient against immunisation by C and E antigens. When Rh 'positive' (C positive and/or E positive) but D-negative blood donors, on admission to hospital, require blood transfusion they deserve a detailed explanation of their blood group and must be transfused with Rh-negative blood. Furthermore, when such female donors become pregnant they should receive prophylaxis for haemolytic disease of the newborn.

D^u antigen and D variants

D^u is a weak form of D antigen; on testing with several anti-D antisera, some will agglutinate D^u red cells whereas others will fail to do so (see also Ch. 19). As blood donors D^u individuals must be grouped as Rh(D) positive. As prospective recipients of blood transfusion D^uindividuals are also grouped as Rh(D) positive and can be transfused safely with Rh(D)-positive blood. However, whenever there is doubt on the basis of

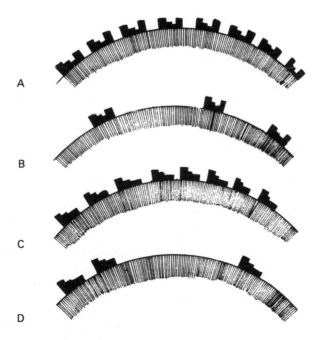

A

B

C

D

Fig. 1.2 Schematic representation of D^u antigen, D variant and D^u variant on the red cell. (A) Normal numbers of antigen sites on the red cell; (B) D^u antigen is qualitatively the same as D antigen, but the number of antigenic sites is reduced; (C) D variant lacks one or several of D antigenic determinants but the number of sites is normal; (D) D^u variant lacks some antigenic determinants and there is a reduced number of sites.

agglutination reactions whether the phenotype is D^u or Rh(D) negative, Rh(D)-negative blood should be transfused. The same policy is applicable to the prevention of haemolytic disease of the newborn in women with D^u antigen. They do not require administration of anti-Rh(D) immunoglobulin unless there is doubt as to whether the phenotype is D^u or Rh(D) negative (see also Ch. 13). *D variants* lack one or more antigenic determinants (epitopes) of the D antigen (Fig. 1.2). They also react with some but not all anti-D antisera. Individuals with D variants can produce antibodies with the specificity of the missing D determinant. However, the administration of anti-Rh(D) immunoglobulin to women with D variant following a pregnancy with a D-positive infant does not seem justifiable in view of the rarity of reports on the production of anti-D in subjects with D variants.

Other Rh antigens
These include C and c, E and e, as well as antigens G (combination of C and D), C^w (related to C), ce, V (variant of ce) and many others.

Red cells lacking Rh antigens
Rarely red cells lack one or more Rh antigens. Rh_{null} is a rare genotype characterised by complete absence of all Rh antigens. In some families Rh_{null} is associated with congenital haemolytic anaemia.

Antibodies of the Rh system

Antibodies of the Rh system are all immune with the exception of some naturally occurring anti-E antibodies.

Anti-D is the most important Rh antibody in clinical blood transfusion. It is invariably immune and causes both haemolytic transfusion reaction and haemolytic disease of the newborn. Anti-D antibodies are invariably detected by the indirect antiglobulin test, and do not bind complement. A few examples of IgM anti-D antibodies which agglutinate untreated red cells in saline have been described. Anti-C may be found together with anti-D antibodies.

Anti-c is the second most important antibody in the Rh system, and can cause haemolytic disease of the newborn as well as immediate and delayed transfusion reactions.

Other Rh antibodies are: anti-C, anti-C^w, anti-E and anti-e. All can cause serious clinical problems, but are encountered much less frequently than the first two antibodies. Autoantibodies with Rh specificity are described on p. 141.

THE KELL SYSTEM

The Kell system is clinically the the third most important blood group system, after the ABO and Rh systems.

Antigens of the Kell system

Genes, gene products and gene frequencies
There are three pairs of allelic genes K and k, Js^a and Js^b and Kp^a and Kp^b. The incidence of K is 0.046, and of k is 0.940. Js^b and Kp^b have a very high frequency like k, whereas Js^a and Kp^a are rare. In exceptionally rare cases with the phenotype K_o, none of the antigens coded by the six genes is expressed on the red cells, and only the precursor substance, K_x antigen, is present on red cells as well as on leucocytes. Individuals lacking K_x on red cells have McLeod syndrome with acanthocytosis and haemolytic anaemia. Some patients also lack K_x antigens on the leucocytes, and they in addition suffer from Type II chronic granulomatous disease.

Genotypes, phenotypes and phenotype frequencies
In Britain genotypes are KK, Kk and kk; 9% of the population are of K-positive phenotype (KK, 0.2% and Kk, 8.7%) and 91% are K-negative. The K-positive phenotype is rarely found in Negroes.

Js^a and Kp^a are rare in Britain, but Js^a is found in 20% of Negroes.

Antibodies of the Kell system

Anti-K is a common antibody since K antigen is highly immunogenic and capable of immunising one out of 10 K-negative recipients of a unit of K-positive blood. Anti-K is an IgG antibody, which can cause haemolytic transfusion reaction and haemolytic disease of the newborn. It is best detected by the antiglobulin test.

Other antibodies
Anti-k, anti-Kp^a, anti-Kp^b, anti-Js^a and anti-Js^b have all been described. The clinical syndromes caused by these antibodies were usually mild. Subjects with McLeod syndrome, when transfused, develop an antibody against the precursor substance K_x. This antibody is called anti-KL and can cause severe transfusion reactions.

THE DUFFY SYSTEM

Antigens of the Duffy system

Genes and gene frequencies
There are allelic genes Fy^a and Fy^b with the incidence of 0.425 and 0.557, respectively; Fy^x with the incidence of 0.016, and the amorphic gene Fy which is very rare in Caucasian populations, but common in Afro-Caribbean people, sometimes reaching the frequency of 1.0.

Genotypes, phenotypes and their frequencies
In the British population there are three common genotypes: Fy^aFy^a, Fy^aFy^b and Fy^bFy^b; Fy^a antigen is present in 66% and Fy^b antigen in 80%

of individuals. Over 80% of Negroes have phenotype Fy(a−b−) which is presumed to provide resistance to infection with *P.vivax* malaria.

Antibodies of the Duffy system

*Anti-Fy*ᵃ is an immune antibody. It is three times less frequent than anti-K; nevertheless, it is frequently implicated in haemolytic transfusion reactions and can cause severe haemolytic disease of the newborn. Anti-Fyᵃ is detected only by the antiglobulin test. *Anti-Fy*ᵇ is very rare.

THE KIDD SYSTEM

Antigens of the Kidd system

Genes and gene frequencies
The genes are allelic, *Jk*ᵃ and *Jk*ᵇ, with the frequency of 0.514 and 0.486, respectively.

Genotypes, phenotypes and their frequencies
In the white races there are three common genotypes, *Jk*ᵃ*Jk*ᵃ, *Jk*ᵃ*Jk*ᵇ, and *Jk*ᵇ*Jk*ᵇ with frequencies of 0.26, 0.50 and 0.24, respectively. Thus 76% of people have Jkᵃ antigen and 74% have Jkᵇ antigen. In the Far East the phenotype Jk(a−b−) has been noted.

Antibodies of the Kidd system

*Anti-Jk*ᵃ and *anti-Jk*ᵇ are invariably immune antibodies and usually found in multitransfused patients. Both antibodies are known to cause haemolytic transfusion reaction and haemolytic disease of the newborn. They are both detected by the antiglobulin test.

THE LUTHERAN SYSTEM

Antigens of the Lutheran system

Genes and gene frequencies
The genes are allelic, *Lu*ᵃ and *Lu*ᵇ, with frequencies of 0.039 and 0.961, respectively.

Genotypes, phenotypes and their frequencies
There are three genotypes *Lu*ᵃ*Lu*ᵃ (0.15%),*Lu*ᵃ*Lu*ᵇ (8%) and *Lu*ᵇ*Lu*ᵇ(92%). A rare phenotype Lu(a−b−) has also been described. Most people who are Lu(a+) have genotype *Lu*ᵃ*Lu*ᵇ.

Antibodies of the Lutheran system

Anti-Lu^a can be naturally occurring or immune, and neither antibody has been clearly implicated in haemolytic transfusion reaction or in haemolytic disease of the newborn. Anti-Lu^b is an exceptionally rare immune antibody and has caused a mild delayed haemolytic transfusion reaction. Both antibodies are usually in part IgM immunoglobulins, agglutinate red cells suspended in saline and react best at 20°C.

THE MNSs SYSTEM

Antigens of the MNSs system

Genes, gene products and gene frequencies
There are two pairs of allelic genes *M* and *N*, and *S* and *s*, which are closely related. *M* and *N* determine the terminal amino acid sequence of glycophorin A (a red cell membrane protein) and *S* and *s* that of glycophorin B. The haplotype* frequencies are: *MS*, 0.247; *Ms*, 0.283; *NS*, 0.080; *Ns*, 0.390.

Genotypes, phenotypes and their frequencies
There are three genotypes, *MM*, *MN* and *NN* with frequencies of 28, 50 and 22%, respectively. The corresponding phenotypes are MM, MN, and NN. Among the British 78% possess antigen M and 70% possess antigen N; 55% have phenotype S and 89% phenotype s. There are many rare genetic variants associated with the MNSs system, including a complete absence of MN glycoprotein (En(a−) cells); or, the presence of the rare allele of *S* and *s*, *S^u*. Individuals homozygous for *S^u* lack both S and s antigens and the common antigen U, and are called U−. This phenotype is relatively common in Negroes (about 1% incidence).

Antibodies of the MNSs system

Anti-M is a relatively rare antibody, usually a cold agglutinin but some warm reacting antibodies have been described. It can cause haemolytic transfusion reaction and haemolytic disease of the newborn, but both syndromes are rare.

Anti-N antibody is extremely rare. However, a high proportion of patients undergoing renal dialysis with reusable membrane filters sterilised by formaldehyde may develop the anti-Nf antibody due to the exposure of red cells, residual in the filter, to formaldehyde. *Anti-S, anti-s* and *anti-U* are common antibodies, usually immune. All three have caused haemolytic transfusion reaction and, very rarely, haemolytic disease of the newborn.

* A haplotype is a segment on chromosome with two or more closely linked loci.

OTHER SYSTEMS OF RED CELL ANTIGENS

Other systems of red cell antigens are *Diego, Cartwright, Xg, Dombrock, Scianna* and *Sid*. The genes, genotypes, phenotypes and their frequencies are shown in Table 1.11. The clinical importance of these systems is limited, because the antibodies are extremely rare. However, when such antibodies occur in a patient, there may be serious difficulties in collecting the right type of blood for transfusion.

The Wright system of antigens is coded by genes Wr^a and Wr^b. The incidence of Wr^a is 0.001, and most people are homozygous for Wr^b. Naturally occurring anti-Wr^a antibody is found in 1% of blood samples. For autoantibodies with anti-Wr^a specificity see p. 141.

Many other, low incidence or high incidence antigens with corresponding antibodies have been described as causes of haemolytic transfusion reaction or mild forms of haemolytic disease of the newborn.

Table 1.11 Genes, genotypes, phenotypes and their frequencies for some clinically less important blood group systems

System	Genes	Gene frequency	Genotype or phenotype	Genotype frequency %	Comment
Diego	Di^a		Di(a+)	0	in Whites
				35	in South American Indians
				5–15	in Chinese and Japanese
	Di^b	1.00	Di(b+)	100	in Whites
Cartwright	Yt^a	0.959	Yt(a+b−)	91.9	
	Yt^b	0.041	Yt(a+b+)	7.9	
			Yt(a−b+)	0.2	
Xg	Xg^a	0.659	Xg(a+)	70 males	
	Xg^*	0.341	Xg(a−)	90 females	
			Xg^a	70 males	
			Xg^aXg^a	43.4	
			Xg^aXg	45.0	in females
			$XgXg$	11.6	
Dombrock	Do^a	0.42	Do(a+)	66	
	Do^b	0.58	Do(b+)	82	
Colton	Co^a	0.959	Co(a+)	99.8	
	Co^b	0.041	Co(b+)	8	
			Co(a+b−)	90.5	
			Co(a+b+)	9.0	
			Co(a−b+)	0.5	
Scianna	Sc^1	0.992	Sc:−1	1 in 10 000	high frequency antigen
	Sc^2	0.008	Sc:2	1	low frequency antigen
Sid	Sd^a		Sd(a+)	91	English population
			Sd(a−)	4	
	Cad				very strong form of Sd^a
Wright	Wr^a	0.001			
	Wr^b				most people are homozygous for Wr^b

* *Xg* is a postulated silent gene.

REFERENCES

Hoffbrand A V, Lewis S M (ed) 1981 Postgraduate haematology, 2nd edn. Heinemann, London

Issit P D, Issit C H 1975 Applied blood group serology, 2nd edn. Spectra Biologicals, Oxnard, California

Mollison P L 1983 Blood transfusion in clinical medicine, 7th edn. Blackwell Scientific, Oxford

Petz L D, Swisher S N (ed) 1981 Clinical practice of blood transfusion. Churchill Livingstone, New York

Race R R, Sanger R 1975 Blood groups in man, 6th edn. Blackwell Scientific, Oxford

Stroup M, Treacy M 1982 Blood group antigens and antibodies. Ortho Diagnostic, Raritan, New Jersey

2. WHOLE BLOOD AND PREPARATIONS OF RED CELLS

Whole blood and red cell preparations are administered to the patient as 'units', a unit being the quantity taken at one time from a blood donor. However, there is a considerable variation in the content of each unit for the following reasons: individual variability of the donors, volume of blood collected, processing of blood into components which is sometimes associated with a loss of cellular elements and/or plasma, and the length of storage. The extent of the variation of the volume of red cells in a unit of blood is shown on Table 2.1.

Table 2.1 The range for red cell volume in a unit of blood

PCV of the donor's blood, l/l*	0.38–0.50
Volume of blood collected, ml**	405–495
Volume of anticoagulant (CPD or CPDA−1)†, ml	63
Total volume of blood in the unit, ml	468–558
Red cell volume in the unit, ml	154–248

* Lower limit for the normal range for women and upper limit of the normal range for men
** Average volume of blood collected is 450 ml with the acceptable variation of ± 10%
† Volume of ACD anticoagulant: 73 ml

The properties of whole blood depend also on the type of anticoagulant used for collection of blood and on the procedures for separation of cellular components and plasma, either shortly after the collection, or later, immediately prior to administration to the patient (Table 2.2). The properties of whole blood and red cell preparations also depend on the length of storage. With time there is a loss of function of some blood constituents and accumulation of harmful bioactive constituents (p. 21, 105, 107).

WHOLE BLOOD

Definition
Blood collected into an anticoagulant/preservative solution in a suitable container and not processed in any manner. It contains all the cellular and plasma constituents of blood, subject to changes on storage, with the exception of ionisable calcium which is precipitated by citric acid, present in citrate containing anticoagulants.

Properties
The volume of blood is usually 450 ml taken into 75 ml of ACD or 63 ml

Table 2.2 Properties of whole blood and blood components depend on the type of anticoagulant and separation of cellular components and plasma

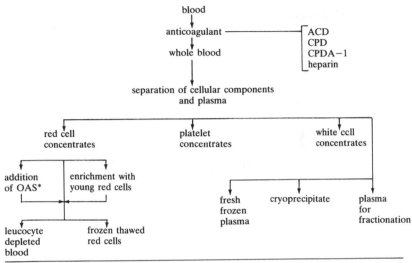

*OAS: Optimal additive solution (see p. 25)

of CPD or CPDA-1 anticoagulant solution. The properties of whole blood depend on the anticoagulant used and on the duration of storage. It should be noted that the anticoagulant solution dilutes the plasma by about 20%.

Storage
Blood is stored at 4 to 8°C. The following changes take place during storage.

1. *Red cells* rapidly lose ATP and 2,3-DPG on storage. The loss of ATP depends partly on the anticoagulant solution used for collecting blood. For example the addition of adenine to the CPD solution has extended the shelf-life* of blood from 28 to 35 days.

   The concentration of 2,3-DPG also falls with time and at a faster rate than that of ATP. However, once transfused, the red cells restore their concentration of 2,3-DPG in about 24 hours. The clinical significance of the reduction in 2,3-DPG in stored blood is uncertain. Fresh blood will provide the optimum concentration of 2,3-DPG. Further details are given in Table 2.3.

2. *White cells.* Granulocytes begin to lose their phagocytic and bactericidal properties within four to six hours of collection

* Shelf-life is defined as the time of storage after which, after transfusion, at least 70% of transfused red cells remain in the recipient's circulation.

Table 2.3 Red cell changes on storage in the blood collected in CPD

Property	Days of storage				
	0	7	14	21	28
Packed cell volume, l/l	0.363	0.358	0.365	0.347	0.357
Red cell 2,3-DPG, %	100	99	50	15	5
Red cell ATP, %	100	96	83	86	75
Survival of red cells after transfusion, %	100	98	85	80	75

Modified from Blood component therapy. A physician's handbook 1981

and they are deemed to be non-functional after 24 hours of storage. However, granulocytes do not lose their antigenic properties. They are capable of sensitising the recipient and causing non-haemolytic febrile transfusion reaction in the immunised recipient. Some viable lymphocytes may be found even after three weeks of storage.

3. *Platelets* lose their haemostatic functions within 48 hours in whole blood stored at 4°C.
4. *Coagulation factors* V and VIII and to a lesser extent XI, rapidly lose their coagulant activity and there is less than 50% of the initial activity within 48 to 72 hours of storage. Thereafter, the rate of loss of clotting activity is less rapid.
5. *Biochemical changes* in stored blood are shown on Table 2.4.
6. *Microaggregates* Aggregates of aged platelets, leucocytes, fibrin strands, cold-insoluble globulin and cellular debris are formed on storage. Their number and size increase proportionally to the duration of storage. Microaggregates pass through the filter of the administration set, but can be removed by in-line microaggregate filters (p. 26).

Table 2.4 Biochemical changes which occur on storage of whole blood collected in CPD

Plasma constituent	Days of storage				
	0	7	14	21	28
pH	7.20	7.00	6.89	6.84	6.78
Oxygen P_{50}, mmHg	23.5	23.0	20.0	17.0	17.0
Sodium, mEq/l	168	166	163	156	154
Potassium, mEq/l	3.9	11.9	17.2	21.0	22.5
Glucose, mg/dl	345	312	282	231	230
Inorganic phosphate, PO_4 mM/l	3.6	3.6	4.2	4.9	5.5
Haemoglobin, mg/dl	1.7	7.8	12.5	19.1	28.9

Modified from Blood component therapy. A physician's handbook 1981

Indications for use
Whole blood is used for patients who require both the replacement of red cells and their oxygen carrying capacity, and the restoration of the circulatory volume. Note that stored whole blood has defective haemostatic properties and if these are required fresh-frozen plasma should be transfused in addition to whole blood.

Whole blood, cryoprecipitate removed

Definition
Whole blood reconstituted with plasma after the removal of
cryoprecipitate.
Properties are essentially the same as for whole blood, except that the
volume of plasma is about 20 ml less and that the unit contains little or
no factor VIII and about half of the initial amount of fibrinogen.
Indications for use are as for whole blood.

Whole blood, platelets removed

Definition
Whole blood reconstituted with plasma after the removal of platelets.
Properties are the same as for whole blood, except that the unit
contains little or no platelets.
Indications for use are as for whole blood.

RED CELL CONCENTRATES

Definition
Red cells obtained by removing 200 to 250 ml of plasma following
centrifugation or sedimentation of a unit of blood.

Properties
Red cell concentrates have PCV higher than 0.75 1/1. Other properties of
red cell concentrates are the same as those of whole blood. Although the
reduction of plasma volume does not affect substantially the shelf-life it is
advisable to use red cell concentrates as soon as practical. In some blood
transfusion centres only about 180 ml of plasma is removed from the unit
of whole blood; in this preparation, called '*plasma reduced blood*', the
PCV is 0.55 to 0.65 1/1.

Indications for use
Restoration of the red cell mass in anaemic patients in whom the increase
in the circulatory volume is not required. It is generally better tolerated
than whole blood since the volume transfused is smaller.

FRESH BLOOD

Definition
Whole blood, plasma reduced blood or concentrated red cells less than
one day old. Some blood banks consider blood as fresh for up to two
days.

Properties
Fresh whole blood contains functional platelets and almost normal concentrations of labile coagulation factors, and red cell 2,3-DPG and ATP.

Indications for use are transfusion and exchange transfusion of neonates.

Comment
Stored blood, supplemented with fresh frozen plasma, clotting factor concentrates or platelet concentrates (as the case may be) is an equally good source of coagulation factors and platelets as fresh blood.

HEPARINISED BLOOD

Definition
Blood collected into heparin.

Properties
A unit is 500 ml of blood collected into 30 ml of heparin (2250 i.u.). The anticoagulant effect of heparin depends on the interreaction with antithrombin III and does not involve calcium. The concentration of ionised calcium is normal.

Shelf-life is 24 hours; heparinised blood is therefore always given fresh.

Indications for use
Exchange transfusion and cardio-pulmonary bypass in the neonate.

Comment
Although it is possible to convert blood collected in citrate into heparinised blood (by adding heparin and calcium gluconate) it is hard to find a justifiable reason to do so.

BLOOD ENRICHED WITH YOUNG RED CELLS

Definition
Blood which contains higher than the average proportion of young cells.

Properties
Blood enriched with young red cells is collected using a cell separator or prepared from single units of blood by differential centrifugation. It is fresh, being either immediately available for transfusion or frozen within 24 hours of collection. As considerable numbers of leucocytes are separated together with the young red cells, blood should be made 'leucocyte poor' by filtration or freezing prior to transfusion. The red cell mass in a 'unit' of blood varies from 50 to 200 ml and should be recorded for each unit transfused when evaluating the patient's response to transfusion.

Shelf-life is 24 hours following collection of blood or thawing of red cells.

Indications for use
Blood enriched with young red cells is used for transfusion to patients with severe bone marrow failure and iron overload, which occur for example in thalassaemia major or aplastic anaemia. However, the advantage of using blood enriched with young red cells has not yet been conclusively proven.

RED CELLS SUSPENDED IN OPTIMAL ADDITIVE SOLUTIONS

Definition
Red cells suspended in a special, protein poor, preservative solution.

Properties
Red cells suspended in an optimal additive solution (OAS) are obtained by centrifugation of a unit of blood, removal of plasma and addition of 100 ml of solution containing sodium chloride, glucose, a nucleotide such as adenine, and mannitol*. OAS does not contain protein, the viscosity of the red cell suspension is low and allows fast administration. The use of OAS combines the advantages of achieving maximum harvesting of plasma for fractionation and high rate of acceptance by medical staff.
    Shelf-life of red cells suspended in OAS is five weeks.

Indications for use
Treatment of anaemia in patients who do not require volume replacement or who have lost less than a half of the blood volume.

Precautions
Transfusion of red cells suspended in OAS to patients who have lost more than a half of the blood volume may have to be supplemented by infusions of albumin. Red cells suspended in OAS are not recommended for use in open heart surgery.

Contraindications
1. Red cells suspended in OAS should not be used for transfusion to neonates and infants.
2. Red cells suspended in OAS should not be transfused to anaemic patients with hypoproteinaemia such as patients with liver disease, renal disease or severe burns.

LEUCOCYTE DEPLETED BLOOD

Definition: a unit of blood (or red blood cells) from which at least 70% of leucocytes are removed.

---

* The volume and composition of each of the OASs available on the market varies from one manufacturer to another.

Properties of leucocyte depleted blood depend on the method chosen for leucocyte removal; the following methods are available.

1. *Centrifugation* of blood packs is carried out in an upright position and the plasma and buffy coat removed with a plasma expressor, or in an inverted position and the cells removed by draining into a transfer pack. Using these techniques leucocyte depletion is about 80% and the red cell loss ranges from 10 to 40%. Shelf-life of leucocyte depleted blood is 24 hours.

2. *Washed red cells* Addition of saline to the packed red cells enables the removal of buffy coat to be repeated several times, improving the leucocyte depletion. The procedure can be carried out manually but the use of blood cell processors (Cobe Blood Cell Processor, the Haemonetics systems and the Elutramatic system) is much more convenient. Using the Cobe 2991 Blood Cell Processor one can produce depletion of about 90%, but the efficiency of other systems is less. The loss of red cells may be as high as 20%. Machine red cell washing techniques remove more than 90% of platelets and almost all the plasma. The shelf-life of washed red cells is 24 hours.

3. *Sedimentation* of red cells with high molecular weight polymers (dextran, gelatin and hydroxyethyl starch) is usually done manually. The procedure removes about 90% of leucocytes and over 90% of platelets. The loss of red cells is small, less than 10%. Shelf-life is 24 hours.

   Note that a small amount of the sedimenting agent is administered with the blood, but the amount is too small to affect the recipient's plasma volume. For other reactions to polymers (all of which are rare) see p. 82, 83.

4. *Filtration* of blood can be carried out using 'specific' leucocyte depleting filters or microaggregate filters. *'Specific' leucocyte depleting filters* are capable of removing up to 100% of the leucocytes and 70 to 98% of the platelets. Red cell losses caused by filtration with 'specific' leucocyte depleting filters are on average 10%. Plasma is not removed, unless centrifugation and plasma removal is carried out before and after filtration (Tables 2.5 and 2.6). The shelf-life of filtered blood is 24 hours.

   Microaggregate filters, in widespread use for the prevention of pulmonary microemboli due to microaggregates present in stored whole blood, can also deplete blood of leucocytes. Several types of microaggregate filters are commercially available all of which have a similar capacity to reduce leucocyte numbers in stored blood regardless of whether they are of a screen or depth type. The leucocyte depletion achieved with microaggregate filters is on average 40%, but

Table 2.5 A comparison of methods used for preparation of leucocyte depleted blood

Procedure	Average Depletion, %			Average red cell loss, %	Complexity of procedure	Cost
	Leucocytes	Platelets	Plasma			
Centrifugation	80	80	8	20	simple	inexpensive
Saline washing, machine	85	95	98	15	moderately complex	moderately expensive
Sedimentation	90	95	95	5	moderately complex	inexpensive
Filtration*						
'specific' leucocyte depleting filters	95	90	Nil**	10	moderately complex	moderately expensive
microaggregate filters	40	40	Nil	None	simple	inexpensive
Freezing and thawing of red cells	98	100	100	10	complex	expensive

* The list of filters and their manufacturers is presented in Table 2.6.
** When blood is centrifuged prior to and after centrifugation and the filtered red cells suspended in saline plasma content may be reduced by up to 85%.

Table 2.6 'Specific' leucocyte depleting filters and microaggregate filters

Name of the filter	Manufacturer
'Specific' leucocyte depleting filters	
Cellselect Filter	NPBI BV, Amsterdam, The Netherlands
Erypur Filter	Organon Teknika BV, Oss, The Netherlands
Imugard IG 500 Filter	Ternmo Corporation, Tokyo, Japan
Sepacell R-500	Asahi Medical Co Ltd, Tokyo, Japan
Microaggregate filters	
Bentley PFF-100s	Bentley Laboratories, Irvine, California, USA
Biotest MF 10B	Biotest Serum Institute GmbH Frankfurt, West Germany
Fenwal 4C2131	Fenwal Laboratories, Deerfield, Illinois, USA
Interface Model 30	Medical Inc., Inver Grove, Minnesota, USA
Ultipor SQ 40S	Pall Biomedical Corporation, Glen Cove, New York, USA
Sorenson-Swank ATS F10	Sorenson Research Co, Salt Lake City, Utah, USA
Travenol 4C 2423	Travenol Laboratories Ltd, Thetford, UK

this can be increased to about 55% by centrifugation of blood prior to filtration. Depletion of platelets is also about 40%, and red cell losses are negligible. Microaggregate filters are 'in-line' filters, i.e. connected to the administration set.

5. *Freezing and thawing* consistently produces units of red cells almost entirely depleted of leucocytes. The methods available for freezing and thawing and the cryopreservatives used are described on p. 29. The process removes 98% of leucocytes and platelets and all the plasma. The red cell losses are usually about 10%. Shelf-life is 24 hours after thawing.

6. *Combined techniques*, for example centrifugation and saline washing followed by filtration or freezing and thawing of red cells, can be used to achieve a complete removal of leucocytes. However, the red cell loss can be as high as 40%. This approach to leucocyte depletion of blood is reserved only for exceptional situations.

Indications for use

1. Prevention of non-haemolytic febrile transfusion reaction (NHFTR) caused by antibodies to leucocyte and HLA antigens in sensitised patients receiving multiple transfusions. A small proportion of NHFTR is the result of immunisation against plasma proteins, for example the development of anti-IgA antibody in patients lacking IgA. Such patients should receive red cell suspensions prepared by one of the methods which completely remove the plasma (saline washing or freezing and thawing of red cells).

2. Prevention of sensitisation of potential recipients of tissue transplants who require blood transfusions. For details see Chapter 16.

Selections of methods for leucocyte depletion

For the prevention of NHFTR one should initially use microaggregate filters at the bedside which may be sufficient to abolish NHFTR in many patients. Should this be ineffective in preventing NHFTR, blood should be depleted of leucocytes by filtration with a 'specific' leucocyte depleting filter, saline washing or freezing and thawing.

Although leucocyte depleted blood contains only a few viable lymphocytes, it would be advisable to irradiate it before administration to an immunosuppressed or immunodeficient recipient, thus preventing possible graft versus host disease (p. 97).

FROZEN AND THAWED RED CELLS

Definition

Saline suspension of red cells prepared by freezing and thawing.

Preparation

Freezing of red cells is most commonly carried out using glycerol as cryopreservative. Glycerol can be used at the concentration of 3.8 M with rapid freezing of red cells and storage in liquid nitrogen, or at a higher concentration (6.2 M or 8.6 M) with a slow rate of freezing and storage at $-85°C$ in mechanical freezers. With both methods thawing is rapid, and it must be followed by extensive washing with electrolyte solutions to remove glycerol.

Properties

It is customary to freeze units of fresh blood. Therefore, the red cell 2,3-DPG and ATP content is about the same as that in the fresh blood. The recovery and survival of frozen and thawed red cells transfused to patients are similar to those for fresh blood. Depletion of leucocytes is over 95%, and most of the platelets and plasma are removed. The red cell losses are about 10%. The shelf-life of frozen red cells is three years, but only 24 hours after thawing.

Indications for use

1. *Freezing of rare blood groups* enables long term storage and supply on a regional, national or international basis, of blood for patients with antibodies against high frequency antigens. It also provides means for storage of blood for autotransfusion. Patients awaiting elective surgery who require blood of a 'rare blood group' should be encouraged to donate blood for autotransfusion (p. 43).
2. *Prevention of NHFTR* in patients sensitised to leucocytes, platelets or plasma proteins (p. 96).
3. *Prevention of sensitisation* against HLA antigens in potential recipients of tissue transplants (p. 163).

Note that the decision to transfuse frozen and thawed red cells should be made after discussing the merits of each case with the blood bank because their preparation is time consuming and expensive.

REFERENCES

American Association of Blood Banks, Washington. 1981 Blood components therapy, a physician's handbook, 3rd edn.
Department of Health and Social Security 1984 Notes on transfusion
Department of Health and Social Security 3/1979 Standards for the collection and processing of blood and blood components and the manufacture of associated sterile fluids
Huestis D W, Bove J R, Busch S 1981 Practical blood transfusion. Little, Brown, Boston

3. SPECIAL PROBLEMS IN BLOOD TRANSFUSION

MULTIPLE TRANSFUSIONS

Definition
Repeated transfusions of blood (or red cells) over a long period of time (months or years).

Indications
Replacement of red cells in patients suffering from
1. *absent or defective erythropoiesis* (aplastic anaemia, pure red cell aplasia, refractory dyserythropoietic anaemias, suppression of erythropoiesis by malignant tissue(s) or drugs);
2. *haemolytic anaemias*, chronic and severe (thalassaemia major, sickle cell anaemia, severe PNH, autoimmune haemolytic anaemia);
3. *recurrent episodes of blood loss*, usually from the GI tract and due to diseases not amenable to surgery (oesophageal varices, angiodysplasia, hereditary haemorrhagic telangiectasiae, congenital and acquired platelet abnormalities and vascular diseases).

Blood required
Plasma reduced blood; concentrated red cells for patients with severely impaired cardio-vascular system. *Leucocyte depleted blood* for patients with a history of non-haemolytic febrile transfusion reaction (Ch. 2).

Blood should be of the same ABO and Rh group, and K-negative for K-negative recipients. It is advisable to phenotype the patient before commencing a multiple transfusion programme, but phenotyped blood for transfusion should not be requested. If and when alloantibodies against red cell antigens develop the compatible blood will be provided by the Regional Blood Transfusion Centre.

Usually blood up to ten days old is satisfactory for transfusion since there is no substantial reduction of the red cell life span within that period of time. Methods for collection of blood rich in young cells and indications for its use are described in Chapter 2.

The volume of blood required *in adults* depends on the initial and desired concentrations of haemoglobin. Each unit of blood will raise the haemoglobin concentration by approximately 1 g/dl (the rise may be smaller in patients with splenomegaly). The *frequency* of blood transfusions depends on the rate of haemoglobin fall and the state of the cardio vascular system; elderly patients rarely tolerate haemoglobin concentration of less than 8.0 g/dl without signs of cardiac failure. When erythropoiesis is non-existant or completely ineffective five or six units of blood are required every five to seven weeks.

In children the required volume of red cells to be transfused (V) can be calculated from the formula:

$$V = W \times (PCV_1 - PCV_0)$$

where W is body weight in kg; PCV_0 and PCV_1 are the initial and desired PCV, respectively, expressed as a percentage.

Example: What is the volume of red cells required for a 20 kg child whose haematocrit is 12% and is to rise to 30%? V = 20 × 18 = 360 ml. Each unit contains approximately 180 ml of red cells.

In this case two units of blood or packed cells are required. The requirement may be much higher in children with splenomegaly who may require two to three times the calculated amount.

The *frequency* of transfusion in children and adolescents depends on the concentration of haemoglobin to be maintained. Most children with congenital anaemia are on *high transfusion regimes*, that is, their haemoglobin is maintained above 8.5 g/dl at all times to enable normal growth and development. Sometimes, *hyper-* or *supertransfusion* is used: the haemoglobin concentration is kept over 11.0 g/dl at all times. This completely suppresses erythropoiesis, abolishes the undesirable effects of hyperactive erythropoiesis on bones, liver, and spleen and most importantly prevents increased iron absorption from the gut.

Administration

In adults up to four units of blood may be administered in 24 hours (for details of circulatory overload see Ch. 11). Temperature and pulse rate should be followed half-hourly. For each unit of blood frusemide 20 mg i.v. should be also administered (to adults). When a non-haemolytic febrile reaction is anticipated, e.g. when leucocyte depleted blood is unavailable and the patient has had reactions to whole blood in the past, an antihistamine (chlorpheniramine, Piriton, 10 mg i.m.) should be given prior to transfusion. Some patients have anaphylactoid reactions to blood and these can be prevented by giving hydrocortisone 100 mg i.v.

In children a scalp vein needle or a small butterfly (19 G or 21 G) should be used as it is essential to preserve the veins. Some children are distressed by the procedure and may need a strong sedative (such as chloral) or even general anaesthesia to cover the setting up of transfusion. Ethyl chloride spray to the venepuncture site will lessen the pain of venepuncture.

Adverse reactions
1. *Alloimmunisation to red cell antigens* (p. 85).
2. *Alloimmunisation to white cell and platelet antigens* (p. 95, 98).
3. *Alloimmunisation to serum antigens* (p. 98).
4. *Other allergic and febrile reactions* (p. 99).
5. *Circulatory overload* (p. 102).

6. *Transmission of disease* (p. 110).
7. *Iron overload.* One litre of blood contains 500 mg of iron; the excretion of iron from the body is only about 1 mg daily. Thus numerous transfusions invariably lead to iron overload. Children with thalassaemia major on transfusion regimes are overloaded with iron by the end of the first decade.

Prevention and treatment of iron overload
Desferrioxamine (Desferal) should be given as a slow subcutaneous infusion using a light portable infusion pump (Graseby Dynamics, Bushey, Watford, Herts.). The iron excretion induced by desferrioxamine varies from patient to patient and the optimum dosage and frequency of subcutaneous infusion should be determined for each patient individually. The average daily dose is 1.5–4.0 g over 12 hours four to six times weekly. Desferrioxamine infusions should be started within the first two years of initiating a long term transfusion regime and continued for as long as transfusion is required. Desferrioxamine can also be administered intravenously and intramuscularly. Details of treatment, side effects and evaluation of iron excretion are reviewed by Weatherall & Clegg (1981).

8. *Splenic pooling/hypersplenism* A proprotion of patients on multiple transfusions develop increasing splenomegaly, signs of hypersplenism (thrombocythopenia, neutropenia) and rapidly increasing transfusion requirements. This is particularly common in children with thalassaemia major and adults with myelofibrosis. Most require splenectomy; the decision when to splenectomise must be based on the increase in the spleen size, evidence of hypersplenism, presence of a large red cell pool in the spleen as determined by radio-isotope studies, and increased transfusion requirements (lower than expected haemoglobin increment immediately after the transfusion and shorter interval between transfusions).

9. *Hypertension, convulsions and cerebral haemorrhage* This is a rare syndrome described in association with a high transfusion regime (Wasi et al, 1978). The mortality is high (approximately one third of all patients described died) and the etiology unknown.

Laboratory investigations
Pre- and post-transfusion full blood count is mandatory. Blood samples for other laboratory tests, required for diagnosis and/or management, should be taken *before blood transfusion.*

The time-table for multiple transfusions should be well organized to keep the hospitalisation to a minimum. Admissions should be planned in advance to suit the patient's work pattern or holidays, as well as the hospital and laboratory work schedule. Blood samples for cross-matching should be collected 24 to 48 hours prior to admission, and the cross-matched blood must be available at the time of admission. It is usual to keep patients overnight in the ward and discharge them within 24 hours unless there has been a transfusion reaction.

EXCHANGE TRANSFUSION

Definition
Replacement of the patient's blood by donors' blood. The relationship
between the volume of blood transfused and the proportion of blood
exchanged is shown in Table 3.1. Exchange transfusion in infants differs
from that in adults.

Table 3.1 The relationship between the volume of blood transfused and the proportion of
blood exchanged

Volume of blood transfused (proportion of total blood volume)	Final proportion of the donor blood in the circulation (%)
½	40
1	65
1½	80
2	87
2½	92

Exchange transfusion in infants
The main objectives are: (i) to remove plasma containing alloantibodies
against the infant's red cells (or platelets in neonatal alloimmune
thrombocytopenia); (ii) to replace the infant's red cells with the donor's
cells lacking the corresponding antigen; and/or (iii) to decrease a high
concentration of bilirubin by removing plasma.

Indications
1. *Haemolytic disease of the newborn*, when clinical status, cord
   blood haemoglobin and bilirubin concentrations indicate
   severe disease (Ch. 13).
2. *Jaundice* with a rapid rise of serum bilirubin to over
   300 μmol/l after birth or later during the neonatal period,
   whether as the result of haemolytic disease of the newborn,
   due to exaggerated physiological jaundice, prematurity,
   G-6PD deficiency or other causes.
3. *Neonatal alloimmune thrombocytopenia*, as an adjunct to
   platelet transfusion (Ch. 13).

Blood required
1. Blood should be of an ABO group compatible with both the
   mother and the infant. Rh-negative infants must receive
   Rh-negative blood.
2. It must lack the antigen against which the mother's antibody
   is directed.
3. When blood group O is used for an infant of a different
   ABO group, it should be tested for the presence of high titre
   anti-A and anti-B antibodies. When the tests are not available

or the results are unknown, concentrated red cells should be used.
4. Blood should be as fresh as possible, and never more than two days old.
5. Blood collected in a heparin pack (2250 i.u. of heparin for 500 ml of blood), or in a citrate anticoagulant (ACD, CPD or CPDA-1) can be used for transfusion.
6. Concentrated red cells or frozen-thawed red cells are resuspended in group AB fresh frozen plasma prior to administration.
7. When possible, blood negative for anti-CMV should be transfused to premature and low birth-weight babies.
8. Blood should be compatible when *cross-matched with the mother's serum.*

Volume of blood required for an exchange transfusion is usually one unit. Ideally 200 ml of blood per kg of body weight (three times the total blood volume) should be exchanged, and the minimum acceptable volume is 130 ml of blood per kg body weight (twice the total blood volume).

Administration
A plastic cannula (e.g. umbilical artery catheter, Argyle, 3.5 mm) is passed into the radial vein, umbilical vein, or saphenous vein and 20 to 50 ml aliquots of blood are exchanged. In infants with raised venous pressure who bleed profusely it is safe initially to withdraw more blood than is returned. If a repeated exchange transfusion is considered and the umbilical vein is used, the umbilical stump should be covered with a saline dressing.

Adverse reactions to an exchange transfusion are similar to those seen in a massive blood transfusion of an adult (p. 37–39). The complications of exchange transfusion, related to the site of administration, are: perforation of the umbilical vein, thrombophlebitis of the vein with subsequent portal hypertension and cirrhosis, and necrotizing colitis. In addition infants may suffer from a severe illness when they contract an infection with CMV.

Laboratory investigations
Complete serological investigation (Ch. 19), full blood count and serum bilirubin are required before transfusion, and the latter two tests are repeated post-transfusion. Other tests (platelet count, DIC screening, etc.) are performed when indicated. Note that a sample of blood from the mother must be taken when serological investigation on cord blood is requested. For details see Chapter 13.

Exchange transfusion in adults
The main objective is to replace the abnormal red cells of the patient (e.g. with sickle cell disease) with donors' red cells.
Indications
    1. *Therapeutic exchange transfusion* in severely ill patients

(cerebrovascular accident, bilateral chest syndrome, priapism).

2. *Elective exchange transfusion* at the beginning of a hypertransfusion programme (pregnancy, preparation for major surgery such as total hip replacement).

Blood required is whole blood, plasma reduced blood or concentrated red cells, as fresh as possible, group ABO and Rh compatible, K-negative for K-negative recipients.

Volume of blood used for exchange transfusion is at least twice the patient's blood volume estimated on the basis of body weight (see Appendix I). Blood is exchanged over a period of two to four days if manual exchange is used or in three to four hours with a cell separator. It is safe to 'top up' and to raise the haemoglobin concentration to about 12 g/dl when the percentage of Hb S in the circulation is less than 30%.

Administration
A saline drip should be set up first and at least 1 l of fluid (e.g. 0.5 l sodium chloride 0.9%, 0.5 l dextrose 5% and one to two units of fresh frozen plasma) administered before about 500 ml of blood are withdrawn from the other arm using a butterfly needle or a Venflow catheter and a 50 ml syringe. One unit of warm blood is then transfused over one to two hours. The withdrawal of 500 ml of blood followed by a transfusion of a unit of blood is then repeated twice. It is usually impossible to exchange more than three units of blood in one day; after this is accomplished venesection into a standard blood collection pack can be carried out. The procedure using a cell separator is described on p. 160. Venous access in a severely ill patient is often poor and it is initially impossible or very difficult to use a cell separator.

Elective exchange transfusion is performed in the same manner but venesection using a standard blood collection pack can be carried out from the beginning. Whenever possible the cell separator should be used for elective exchange.

Adverse reactions in addition to those described in Chapters 10 and 11 are:

1. *Immediate*: sludging in the CNS (presenting with drowsiness, headache, acute confusional state or focal neurological signs), or the lungs (presenting with breathlessness and cough). These complications are caused by increased blood viscosity during the early stages of exchange transfusion. It is therefore essential to ensure abundant intravenous fluid input at all times (at least 3 l/m² of body surface in 24 hours).
2. *Late* as in hypertransfusion.

Laboratory investigations
Full blood count and quantitative estimation of Hb S (by electrophoresis on cellulose acetate and scanning or elution) should be carried out before and after exchange transfusion.

MASSIVE TRANSFUSION

Definition
Transfusion of a volume of stored blood, which is greater than the recipient's blood volume, in less than 24 hours.

Indications
Treatment or prevention of hypovolaemic shock caused by profuse bleeding due to a disease, trauma or surgical intervention.

Blood required
Group ABO and Rh compatible, cross-matched, whole blood, plasma reduced blood or red cell concentrates.

Administration
It is advisable to use an in-line microaggregate filter (Ch. 2). When a fast rate of transfusion is required a pressure infusor or a pump and a blood warmer should be used (p. 42).

Other blood components
Transfusion of fresh frozen plasma and platelets may be required (p. 56, 63).

Stored blood contains an excess of citrate, potassium and lactic acid, and lacks ionised calcium, coagulation factors V, VIII:C and XI, functional platelets and granulocytes. It has reduced pH, diminished oxygen-carrying capacity and it is cold (4°C when taken from the storage refrigerator). Therefore, transfusion of a large volume of stored blood may cause the following clinical complications.

Clinical complications
1. *Cardiac abnormalities* are usually ventricular extrasistoles, rarely ventricular fibrillation progressing to cardiac arrest. They are due to the combined effects of low temperature, high potassium concentration, and excess citrate with low calcium concentration.

Prevention and management
A blood warmer should be used when a large volume of blood is transfused within a short period of time (p. 42). Excess of citrate and low calcium concentration become clinically significant only when more than five units of blood are transfused in less than an hour. Calcium gluconate (2 ml of 10% solution per unit of blood) should only be given when calcium concentration in plasma can be monitored. Routine administration of calcium in massive transfusion has not been shown to be beneficial and may even be dangerous. High potassium concentration affects only those recipients with hepatic or renal failure, in whom the rate of transfusion should be reduced.

2. *Acidosis* Low pH of stored blood may aggravate acidosis in the patient with severe renal or liver disease.

Prevention and management
Blood as fresh as possible should be used. Sodium bicarbonate should be

administered after determining the 'base deficit' from the measurements of blood pH and Pco_2. In practice acidosis is rarely a problem, because citrate is metabolised into bicarbonate and produces alkalosis.

3. *Failure of haemostasis* The usual clinical manifestations are failure of local haemostasis and, infrequently, a generalised bleeding tendency due to the lack of factors VIII: C, V and XI, as well as platelets in the stored blood. It occurs when more than twice the blood volume is given, but the very young and some elderly patients with liver disease or rheumatoid arthritis, or those suffering a long period of ill health may show haemostatic abnormalities after only one blood volume has been administered. The diagnosis of bleeding due to massive transfusion must be confirmed by the laboratory, as other haemostatic defects have an identical clinical presentation but require different management. The laboratory investigation and differential diagnosis are presented in Table 3.2.

Table 3.2 Differential diagnosis of haemostatic failure in massive blood transfusion

Condition or disease	LABORATORY TESTS			
	Prothrombin time	Partial thromboplastin time	Thrombin time	Platelet count
Massive blood transfusion	↑	↑	N	↓ [†]
DIC*	↑↑	↑↑	↑↑	↓↓
Vit. K deficiency	↑↑	↑	N	N
Haemophilia	N	↑↑	N	N
ITP**	N	N	N	↓↓

* DIC, disseminated intravascular coagulation
** ITP, idiopathic thrombocytopenic purpura
N normal;
↑ moderately prolonged; ↑↑ markedly prolonged;
↓ moderately decreased; ↓↓ markedly decreased.
[†] Platelet count rarely falls below $50 \times 10^9/l$.

Prevention and management
Fresh frozen plasma, one to two units, corrects the abnormalities of coagulation and should be given prophylactically after every ten units of blood. Platelet transfusion may be required when the platelet count is lower than $30 \times 10^9/l$, particularly if the patient is undergoing a neurosurgical procedure.

4. *Shock lung* or adult respiratory distress syndrome (ARDS) occurs in a severely ill patient after major trauma and/or surgery. A tetrad of clinical features characterises ARDS: progressive respiratory distress, decreased lung compliance, acute hypoxaemia and diffuse radiographic opacification of the lungs. The mortality is high; post mortem studies show widespread macroscopic and microscopic thrombosis in the pulmonary arteries. The pathogenesis of ARDS is unclear, but direct damage to alveolar lining cells, local DIC,

microvascular fluid leakage and embolisation by microaggregates from stored blood (p. 22) all contribute. The use of in-line microaggregate filters to prevent microembolisation is recommended. Platelet transfusion should not be used indiscriminately and if given, a platelet filter must be applied (p. 180).

5. *Jaundice* almost invariably follows massive blood transfusion. However, serum total bilirubin rarely exceeds 40 μmol/l and haemoglobinaemia is slight. Investigation for a delayed haemolytic transfusion reaction is not indicated.

Adverse reactions are as described in Chapters 10 and 11.

Laboratory investigation

Blood samples are collected before and during massive blood transfusion as and when required by the clinical situation

1. *Blood* collected in a *sequestrene tube* is used for haemoglobin determination and platelet count.
2. *Citrated blood* is used for coagulation studies.
3. *Clotted blood* is required for compatibility testing. Note that the transfused blood must be ABO and Rh group compatible if blood of the patient's group is not available. For convenience blood group O and Rh compatible is used. Other blood products, e.g. fresh frozen plasma and platelets should be from the same blood group as the red cells. Also note that with two to three blood volumes replaced there is little point in waiting for the results of urgent crossmatch, as neither plasma nor cells belong to the patient. Nevertheless, compatibility testing must be carried out to detect any (however rare) incompatibility between the units transfused.

TRANSFUSION IN OPEN HEART SURGERY

Definition and indications

Patients undergoing open heart surgery require cardiopulmonary bypass (CPB) for maintaining the circulation with oxygenated blood.

Note that CPB as a part of open heart surgery is a complex procedure and that the demand for blood and blood products is variable in individual patients. It depends on:

1. The total *extracorporeal volume* of the heart-lung machine (for adults it is about 2 l and for children about 1 l), the degree of *haemodilution* desired and the *patient's blood volume*. In adults at the start of CPB it is expected that haemodilution will reduce the red cell count and the concentration of plasma proteins by at least 50%. When a greater degree of haemodilution is required, one or two units of patient's blood can be collected before commencing the CPB, and transfused post-operatively. Note that in infants

and small children blood is required for priming the heart-lung machine.

2. *The type of operation*, e.g. repeated cardiac surgery may become a prolonged procedure with severe blood loss due to multiple adhesions.

3. The degree of *haemostatic defect* in the post-operative period caused by thrombocytopenia, heparin rebound, activation of fibrinolysis or DIC.

4. The patient's initial haematological status, e.g. anaemia, thrombocytopenia or coagulopathy.

5. Personal preferences of the surgeon and/or anaesthetist.

The use of *hypothermia* requires careful testing in the laboratory for the detection of cold antibodies in the patient's blood (Ch. 19).

The blood required should be of the same ABO and Rh group as the patient. Compatibility testing should exclude the presence of cold antibodies in the patient's blood. For *priming* of the heart-lung machine in adults crystalloid solutions (e.g. Hartmann's solution, see p. 83) are used and blood is rarely required for that purpose. In neonates only fresh blood collected in heparin is used. In small children fresh blood collected in heparin is used in preference to the blood collected into citrate. For *post-operative transfusion* in adults citrated whole blood, plasma reduced blood or concentrated red cells are equally satisfactory. Blood only a few days old is preferred to stored blood, but the latter can be used safely. The use of microaggregate filters is advisable when blood stored for several days is transfused.

Volume of blood required for cross-matching in most cases of open-heart procedures is four units. Additional two to four units are required in repeated procedures. Only in exceptional circumstances are more than eight units of blood requested for cross-matching, as for example when the patient is anaemic prior to operation. Neonates and children also require four units of blood (for priming the heart-lung machine). However, the number of units ultimately transfused during the post-operative period varies considerably.

The reduction of body temperature to about 25°C in hypothermia and the use of ice-cold cardioplegic solution during open heart surgery requires a search for cold antibodies and it is advisable to include incubation of 4°C in the compatibility testing. When cold agglutinins are detected their clinical significance must be carefully evaluated, for example weak cold agglutinins with IH specificity can be safely disregarded since they are present in many elderly patients.

Blood components may be required for the correction of the haemostatic defect: fresh frozen plasma, two to four units, administered post-operatively. On rare occasions, platelet count may fall to below 30 $\times$ 10^9/l post-operatively, and then a transfusion of four to eight units of platelets should be given. The use of albumin and PPF either for priming the heart-lung machine or post-operatively has not been proved to be advantageous.

Bleeding associated with CPB is due to:

1. Activation and loss of platelets and coagulation factors in the extracorporeal circulation.
2. Failure of heparin neutralisation by the first dose of protamine.
3. Activation of fibrinolysis in the oxygenator and pump.
4. Disseminated intravascular coagulation in patients with poor cardiac output and long perfusion times.

The differential diagnosis of bleeding associated with CPB is presented in Table 3.3.

Table 3.3 Differential diagnosis of bleeding associated with cardiopulmonary bypass

Cause of bleeding	Prothrombin time	Partial thromboplastin time	Thrombin time without protamin	with protamin	Platelet count
Loss of platelets	N	N	N	N	↓↓
Depletion of coagulation factors	↑↑	↑↑	N	N	N or ↓
Excess of heparin	↑	↑↑	↑	N	N or ↓
Hyper-fibrinolysis	↑	↑	↑↑	↑↑	N or ↓
DIC*	↑↑	↑↑	↑↑	↑↑	↓↓

* DIC, disseminated intravascular coagulation
N normal;   ↑ moderately prolonged;   ↑↑ markedly prolonged;   ↓ moderately reduced;
↓↓ markedly reduced.

Management of bleeding associated with CPB.

1. Thrombocytopenia (platelet count less than $30 \times 10^9/l$) requires administration of four to eight units of platelet concentrates.
2. Loss of coagulation factors is corrected by administration of two to four units of fresh frozen plasma.
3. Excess heparin is neutralised by protamine. The total dose of protamine administered is calculated from the measured plasma heparin concentration, estimated patient's plasma volume and the fact that 1 mg of protamine neutralises approximately 100 i.u. of heparin.
4. Hyperfibrinolysis (if confirmed on laboratory testing) is treated with tranexamic acid i.v. (or a similar antifibrinolytic agent) at the time of diagnosis.
5. Disseminated intravascular coagulation requires in the first instance the correction of the underlying cause (e.g. poor perfusion, oligaemic shock, acidosis, infection, etc.) and then fresh frozen plasma and platelet concentrates as required.

Adverse reactions are the same as those described in Chapters 10 and 11. In addition, increased susceptibility to infection over a period of several weeks after CPB has been noted; the mechanism responsible is not clear. Also patients who received several units of fresh blood are likely to be exposed to infection or reinfection with CMV (Ch. 12).

RAPID TRANSFUSION

Definition
Transfusion of blood at a rate greater than that dependent on gravity (greater than 60 ml/min), under pressure or with a pump.

Indications
Prevention and treatment of oligaemic shock after acute and severe blood loss.

Blood required
Group ABO and Rh compatible, cross-matched. Often rapid transfusion is carried out as an emergency procedure, when there is no time for a cross-match or even the determination of the blood group; then blood group O Rh positive should be used, except for girls and women of reproductive age when O Rh negative blood is used.

Volume of blood required is variable and may reach 50 units or more.

Administration of blood requires an *increased blood* flow which can be achieved by:
1. manual compression and by rolling down a partially empty pack;
2. using a Y-type or a three lead recipient set which enables simultaneous transfusion of two and three units of blood, respectively. Both types of the recipient set are also available with one of the leads fitted with a vent adaptor coupler for single-hole solution bottles;
3. using pressure cuffs from an ordinary blood pressure manometer or a specialised one (Biomed pressor infusor, Fenwal pressure infusor, Tycos pressure infusor);
4. a combination of multiple lead recipient sets with pressure infusors. Using the above techniques a unit fo blood can be given in about two minutes.

In rapid transfusion, blood is usually transfused shortly after being removed from the storage refrigerator and should be *warmed* using an in-line blood warmer (Fenwal Dry Heat Blood Warmer System; the Avon A80 Warming Coil for use with a water bath).

It is advisable to use microaggregate filters whenever several units of blood are transfused (p. 26).

In rapid blood transfusion the use of *blood components, clinical complications, adverse reactions*, and *laboratory investigations* are essentially the same as those described for massive blood transfusion (p. 37–39).

Note that the decision to stop a rapid blood transfusion whether because of its success or failure should be communicated immediately to the hospital blood transfusion laboratory to prevent further efforts to transfer blood from the Regional Blood Transfusion Centre and/or other hospitals.

AUTOLOGOUS TRANSFUSION

Definition
The administration of the patient's own blood collected previously or during an operation.

Indications
1. Provision of blood for the patient with antibodies to one of the hight frequency red cell antigens (public antigens) who is awaiting elective surgery and for whom it is not possible to obtain compatible blood.
2. Provision of blood for recipients who wish to avoid the risks of random donor blood (alloimmunisation, infection), or as an attempt to improve blood supply.
3. Haemodilution prior to surgery; it is used to reduce blood viscosity, enhance blood flow and prevent intravascular thrombosis.
4. Salvage of blood lost due to acute haemorrhage in major surgery and return to the patient.

Procedures employed for autologous transfusion depend on the indications.

1 & 2. Planning the collection of blood from the patient awaiting surgery should take account of the volume required and of the time available. It is possible to collect one unit of blood a week from a patient with normal erythropoiesis and on iron supplements; up to five units can be collected and stored during a five-week period (shelf life of blood collected into CPDA-1 anticoagulant). When more than five units are required or when the patient cannot tolerate frequent donations, either freezing of red cells or the method of 'leap-frogging' may be used. In 'leap-frogging' the first unit of blood collected and sometimes one or two units collected later, is transfused to the patient, so that a fresh unit(s) of blood can be collected and stored.
3. Haemodiluation is performed by withdrawing one or two units of blood from the patient within 24 hours or immediately before an operation; the blood is returned after the operation. Haemodilution is almost always used for open heart surgery and less commonly in other surgical procedures (Urbanyi et al, 1983).
4. Salvage of blood lost in acute haemorrhage is achieved by using a cell saver (Haemonetics Cell Saver III or Cell Saver IV). Blood shed into the thoracic or abdominal cavity is aspirated, the red cells are washed by centrifugation, suspended in saline and transfused to the patient. The use of a cell saver may considerably reduce the number of units

required for transfusion. Contraindications are: blood exposed to a site of infection or the possibility of contamination with malignant cells.

REFERENCES

American Association of Blood Banks, Washington 1981 Blood component therapy, a physician's handbook, 3rd edn

American Association of Blood Banks, Washington 1981 Technical manual of the American Association of Blood Banks, 8th edn

Boggis C R, Greene R 1983 Adult respiratory distress syndrome. British Journal of Hospital Medicine (February): 167–174

Department of Health and Social Security 1984 Notes on transfusion

Plapp F V, Beck M L 1984 Transfusion support in the management of immune naemolytic disorders. In: Bayer W L (ed) Blood transfusion and blood banking. Clinics in Haematology 13: 167–183

Swisher S N, Petz L D 1981 Autologous blood transfusion and blood salvage. In: Petz L D, Swisher S N (eds) Clinical practice of blood transfusion. Churchill Livingstone, Edinburgh

Urbanyi B, Spillner G, Breymann T, Kameda T 1983 Autotransfusion with hemodilution in vascular surgery. International Surgery 68: 37–40

Wasi P, Na-Nakorn S, Pootrakul P, Sonakul D, Piankijagum A, Pacharee P 1978 A syndrome of hypertension, convulsion, and cerebral haemorrhage in thalassaemic patients after multiple blood transfusions. Lancet 2: 602–604

Weatherall D J, Clegg J B 1981 Thalassaemia Syndromes, 3rd edn. Blackwell Scientific, Oxford, ch 6, p 156–162 and ch 13, p 683–743

Zipursky A 1981 Isoimmune haemolytic disease. In: Nathan D G, Oski F A (eds) Hematology of infancy and childhood, 2nd edn. Saunders, Philadelphia, ch 3, p 50–85

4. LEUCOCYTE AND PLATELET ANTIGENS, ANTIGENIC DETERMINANTS ON PLASMA PROTEINS, AND CORRESPONDING ANTIBODIES

Almost all the cells in the body carry numerous antigenic determinants. Two systems of antigens, the ABO and the major histocompatibility system (HLA system), with few exceptions, are common to all cells. In addition to these, red cells, granulocytes, lymphocytes, and platelets each possess specific antigens, which they do not share with other cells. Also there are well defined antigenic determinants on a number of plasma proteins, some of which are important in the practice of blood transfusion.

THE HLA SYSTEM

The HLA system is a single, complex and highly polymorphic system of antigens expressed on leucocytes, platelets and other nucleated cells. Antibodies to the HLA antigens are easily formed and they are of considerable importance in blood transfusion and organ transplantation.

The HLA region is situated on the short arm of chromosome 6 and consists of at least four loci: A, B, C and D. *HLA A, B and C* loci contain genes whose products are class I antigens, cell surface antigens which occur on all nucleated cells. HLA A, B and C antigens are glycoproteins composed of a heavy chain (mw 43 000 daltons), which carries the antigenic specificity, and a light chain (mw 12 000 daltons), β_2-microglobulin. The light chain is coded for on chromosome 15.

The HLA D locus encompasses several different subtypes of antigen: HLA-DR, HLA-DQ, HLA-DP. Their expression is restricted to B lymphocytes, macrophages, vascular endothelial cells, dendritic cells and activated T-lymphocytes. HLA-D locus antigens, or class II antigens are cell surface glycoproteins which play an important role in the regulation of immune process. β_2-microglobulin is not a part of class II antigens.

Each locus of the HLA system can be occupied by one of the many alleles shown on Table 4.1. The specificity of each allele is denoted with

Table 4.1 Antigens of the HLA system
Agreed following the Ninth International Histocompatibility Workshop (1984)

HLA-A	HLA-B	HLA-B	HLA-C
A1	B5	Bw48	Cw1
A2	B7	B49 (21)	Cw2
A3	B8	Bw50 (21)	Cw3
A9	B12	B51 (5)	Cw4
A10	B13	Bw52 (5)	Cw5
A11	B14	Bw53	Cw6
Aw19	B15	Bw54 (w22)	Cw7
A23 (9)*	B16	Bw55 (w22)	Cw8
A24 (9)	B17	Bw56 (w22)	
A25 (10)	B18	Bw57 (17)	
A26 (10)	B21	Bw58 (17)	
A28	Bw22	Bw59	
A29 (w19)	B27	Bw60 (40)	
A30 (w19)	B35	Bw61 (40)	
A31 (w19)	B37	Bw62 (15)	
A32 (w19)	B38 (16)	Bw63 (15)	
Aw33 (w19)	B39 (16)	Bw64 (14)	
Aw34 (10)	B40	Bw65 (14)	
Aw36	Bw41	Bw67	
Aw43	Bw42	Bw70	
Aw66 (10)	B44 (12)	Bw71 (w70)	
Aw68 (28)	B45 (12)	Bw72 (w70)	
Aw69 (28)	Bw46	Bw73	
	Bw47		
	Bw4	broad specific antigens	
	Bw6		

HLA-D	HLA-DR	HLA-DQ	HLA-DP
Dw1	DR1	DQw1	DPw1
Dw2	DR2	DQw2	DPw2
Dw3	DR3	DQw3	DPw3
Dw4	DR4		DPw4
Dw5	DR5		DPw5
Dw6	Drw6		DPw6
Dw7	DR7		
Dw8	DRw8		
Dw9	DRw9		
Dw10	DRw10		
Dw11 (w7)	DRw11 (5)		
Dw12	DRw12 (5)		
Dw13	DRw13 (w6)		
Dw14	DRw52		
Dw15	DRw53		
Dw16			
Dw17 (w7)			
Dw18 (w6)			
Dw19 (w6)			

* Previous specificity is given in brackets.
  Reproduced with permission of Biotest Serum Institut GMBH, Dreieich, West Germany

a number agreed following the Ninth International Histocompatibility Workshop (1984). The letter w indicates a provisional (w, workshop) specificity.

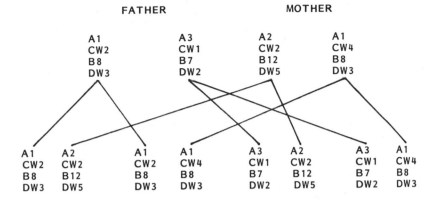

Fig. 4.1 Inheritance of HLA haplotypes. Each child inherits one haplotype from the father and one from the mother.

Inheritance

The HLA genes are closely linked, and inherited as a haplotype (Fig. 4.1). The two haplotypes constitute the HLA genotype of an individual. Within a family the chance that any one sibling is identical to another is 25%. However, with so many alleles at each locus, the chance of finding an identical HLA genotype outside the family is very small.

Geographic and ethnic distribution

Northern Europeans commonly have HLA A1, A3, B7 and B8 antigens. The incidence of B5 and Bw35 increases from the North to the South of Europe. African Negroes have antigens Aw36 and Bw42 which do not occur in other populations; antigen B17 is also frequent in that ethnic group. In Mongol races the antigens with high frequencies are A9, Bw40 and Bw22; antigens A1, A3, B7 and B8 are absent. Antigen A2 is found in all races.

Antibodies to HLA antigens develop following a pregnancy in up to 20% of women and following multiple transfusions in over 50% of recipients. HLA antibodies are responsible for non-haemolytic febrile transfusion reactions in multitransfused patients (p. 96), for refractoriness of platelets in thrombocytopenic patients who have received platelet transfusions in the past (p. 57), and for graft-versus-host disease and transplant rejection in recipients of organ transplants (p. 163).

HLA typing and detection of HLA antibodies

1. Serological typing of HLA A, B and C alleles is carried out using microlymphyocytotoxicity tests. A purified lymphocyte suspension from the individual to be tested is incubated with

antisera of known specificity. The cells reacting with the antiserum, that is having the corresponding antigen on their surface, will be damaged and will take up the dye which is added at the end of incubation.

2. Typing for HLA D alleles is carried out using mixed lymphocyte culture reaction or serological typing. In mixed lymphocyte culture reaction, lymphocytes from the individual to be tested are mixed with lymphocytes of known D specificity in tissue culture. Lymphocytes which are HLA D identical show no response, but lymphocytes which are not identical will undergo transformation and will proliferate. The degree of response is measured by the incorporation of radioactive thymidine into the proliferating cells.

3. Serological typing is carried out for DR alleles using a modified lymphocytotoxicity test. The lymphocyte suspension is enriched in B cells using one of several techniques available and the standard lymphocytotoxicity test is carried out.

4. Detection of anti-HLA antibodies is serum is performed using several tests. *The lymphocytotoxicity test* is most commonly used; the patient's serum is incubated with lymphocytes of known HLA specificity. *The leucocyte agglutination test* is used to detect potent anti-HLA antibodies (see below); the patient's serum is incubated with leucocytes of known specificity, and in the presence of the corresponding antibody the leucocyte suspension will show agglutination under the microscope. Tests with *fluorescein-labelled antiglobulin serum* can also be carried out; a purified suspension of granulocytes is treated with paraformaldehyde to abolish non-specific fluorescence, granulocytes are incubated in the serum containing the specific antibody, and then washed. Finally, the granulocytes are incubated with fluorescein-labelled anti-IgG; if an antibody has been bound to granulocytes, anti-IgG will react with it and show up as fluorescence.

GRANULOCYTE ANTIGENS

Neutrophil antigens (NA) are found exclusively on mature neutrophil granulocytes. They are called NA1 and NA2, NB1, ND1 and NE1. In addition, antigens HGA−1, −2 and −3 are shared with monocytes. Antibodies to these antigens arise as a result of immunisation by pregnancy or transfusion. Rare causes of neonatal alloimmune neutropenia are caused by the presence of antibodies in the mother's circulation to granulocyte antigens.

Typing of granulocytes and detection of antibodies to granulocyte antigens is carried out using the leucocyte agglutination test or fluorescein-labelled antiglobulin serum.

LYMPHOCYTE ANTIGENS

Subsets of lymphocytes with specific surface antigens (markers) have been identified using a number of monoclonal antibodies. Whilst these are of interest in diagnostic haematology they seem to have little importance in blood transfusion.

PLATELET ANTIGENS

Although sensitisation to HLA antigens and HLA antibodies is responsible for most cases of refractoriness to platelet transfusions, antibodies to platelet antigens may also be responsible. However, antibodies to platelet antigens are almost invariably implicated in neonatal alloimmune thrombocytopenia (p. 135) and post-transfusion purpura (p. 146).

Platelet antigens Pl^{A1} and Pl^{A2} are antigenic determinants associated with platelet membrane glycoproteins. The incidence of Pl^{A1} positive and Pl^{A2} positive phenotypes is 98% and 26%, respectively. Bak^a is a platelet antigen present in over 90% of normal people. Other platelet specific antigens are Ko^a, Ko^b, Pl^{E1}, Pl^{E2} and Duzo. Patients with Glanzmann's disease lack platelet membrane glycoproteins IIIa and IIb and also lack Pl^{A1}, Pl^{A2} and Bak^a antigens.

Antibodies to platelet antigens
Anti-Pl^{A1} has been found in almost all cases of alloimmune neonatal thrombocytopenia and post-transfusion purpura, whereas anti-Bak^a and anti-Duzo have been demonstrated in a few cases only. The clinical significance of antibodies against other platelet antigens is uncertain.

Identification of platelet specific antigens and antibodies is carried out using platelet agglutination techniques, either direct or with a fluorescein-labelled antiglobulin serum.

Platelet cross-match has been recently introduced with the aim of selecting compatible platelets for transfusion to patients who have no platelet increment following transfusion of random platelet concentrates (p. 58). The platelet immunofluorescent test (PIFT) is commonly used, in which the donor's platelets and recipient's serum are incubated together; the platelets are then washed and tested with fluorescein-labelled anti-IgG serum. Incompatible platelets show strong fluorescence. A platelet cross-match is helpful when HLA matched platelet concentrates are not available or when there is a poor post-transfusion recovery of HLA matched platelets. Management of platelet refractoriness is described on p. 57.

ANTIGENIC DETERMINANTS ON PLASMA PROTEINS

Plasma proteins carry many antigenic determinants, but there are relatively few antibodies to these determinants which are relevant to blood transfusion.

Antibodies to antigens on IgG

Antibodies are directed either against determinants on the native IgG molecule (Gm system of antigens) or against determinants exposed during the antigen-antibody reaction (anti-antibodies).

Gm determinants are found on the heavy chain of IgG molecules. Anti-Gm may be found in a small proportion of healthy people, usually in women who have been pregnant, or in individuals transfused in the past. Patients with rheumatoid arthritis often possess an autoantibody with anti-Gm specificity in the plasma.

Antibodies to IgA

IgA deficiency is found in about one in 3000 normal people. Such 'deficient' individuals may exhibit a complete lack of IgA or have a selective deficiency of certain subclasses of IgA. These individuals may become immunised to IgA when pregnant or following transfusion. The anti-IgA may give rise to a severe allergic reaction with each subsequent transfusion of blood or plasma.

Antibodies to IgM

are rare. They are usually found in immunodeficient patients.

Antibodies to factor VIII:C and other coagulation factors

Some 7% of patients with haemophilia develop an antibody to factor VIII:C. This antibody is of restricted specificity and does not cause an anaphylactoid reaction, but destroys factor VIII:C in vivo and in vitro Antibodies to other clotting factors have also been described: they all are capable of causing inactivation of the corresponding clotting factor, often associated with severe bleeding.

REFERENCES

Genetet B, Mannoni P 1978 La transfusion. Flammarion Médecine-Sciences, Paris
Mollison P L 1983 Blood transfusion in clinical medicine, 7th edn. Blackwell Scientific, Oxford
Yunis E J, Dupont B 1981 The HLA system. In: Nathan D G, Oski F A (eds) Hematology of
    infancy and childhood, 2nd edn. Saunders, Philadelphia, ch 41, p 1438–1458

5. PLATELET TRANSFUSION

Platelet therapy has been an integral part of treatment in haematological malignancies, especially of acute leukaemia, and has contributed to the improved outlook for many such patients. The increasing demand for platelet concentrates has led the transfusion services to develop new techniques for platelet harvesting and to establish guidelines for the use of concentrates.

PLATELET CONCENTRATES

Methods of collection

Platelet concentrates can be prepared manually or by using a blood cell processor; they can be obtained from a single donor or pooled from several donors; and they can be collected from random donors or from HLA matched or Pl^{A1}-negative donors (Tables 5.1 and 5.2).

Manually prepared platelet concentrates are available as single platelet concentrates harvested from one unit of blood or as pooled platelet concentrates harvested from four to six units of blood. They are prepared from blood collected into a double or triple pack with ACD, CPD or CPDA-1 anticoagulant, as soon as possible after donation and before the blood is refrigerated.

Packs with platelet concentrates are stored at 20° to 24°, preferably in an incubator, on a horizontal, vertical or angled agitator for up to three days. Special platelet packs made of polyolefin enable better aeration of

Table 5.1 Description of platelet concentrates according to the selection of donors and methods of collection

Type of platelet concentrate (PC)	Donor	Method of preparation	Matching process
Random multiple donor PC	random	manual	—
Pooled random multiple donor PC	random	manual	—
Cross-matched random multiple donor PC	random	manual	cross-matched
Random single donor PC	random	cell separator	—
Cross-matched random single donor PC	random	cell separator	cross-matched
HLA typed single donor PC	HLA type selected	cell separator	HLA typed

platelets and extend the shelf life to five days. Alternatively platelet concentrates can be stored at 4° to 6° without mixing for up to three days.

Platelet concentrates obtained by platelet apheresis from a single donor have properties which depend on the type of blood cell processor, anticoagulant, and the protocol used for harvesting (p. 156). The

Table 5.2 Characteristics of platelet concentrates

Characteristic	Method of collection	
	Manual	Cell separator
Volume, ml	50–70	20–500
Platelet content, × 10^{11}	0.5–1.1	2.0–6.0
Red cell content	negligible	may be considerable*
Leucocyte content	negligible	may be considerable*
Storage temperature	20–24°C**	
Agitation	required	
Shelf-life	3 days†	1 day
Recovery 1 h after transfusion, %‡	50–80	
Half-life in circulation‡	4 days	
Main potential risk	bacterial contamination	circulatory overload
Main advantage	good survival	suitable for special preparations (HLA-typed, Pl^{A1}-negative)
Cost	low	high

* May require further processing
** Concentrates stored at 4° C do not require agitation, but have a shorter half-life in circulation and are less haemostatically effective.
† Concentrates stored in polyolefin packs have a shelf life of five days.
‡ Depends on spleen size, presence of infection, bleeding etc.

protocol used will also determine the red cell and leucocyte contamination of the final product. High content of red cells in platelet concentrates may requires cross-matching before transfusion and will require that the concentrates are ABO and Rh group compatible. A high content of leucocytes in platelet concentrates may cause non-haemolytic transfusion reactions which often require treatment (or prophylaxis) with chlorpheniramine (Piriton) and/or hydrocortisone.

HLA matched and Pl^{A1}-negative platelet concentrates are usually prepared by platelet apheresis for a named patient with a clear need for such a preparation. *Washed platelets, leucocyte depleted* and *irradiated* platelet concentrates can be prepared on demand in some transfusion centres.

Frozen and thawed platelets
Platelet concentrates can be frozen in dimethylsulphoxide (DMSO) or glycerol and stored at −150°C or −80°C, respectively, for up to three

years. The techniques used at present give relatively low yields after thawing, but platelet freezing may become an important technique of platelet preservation in the future.

Platelet recovery and survival

The recovery of platelets one hour after transfusion in healthy volunteers is approximately 65%. Nearly one third of the transfused platelets are sequestered in the normal spleen. Splenic sequestration may be much higher in individuals with splenomegaly. The survival of fresh ^{51}Cr labelled autologous platelets is on average nine days, whereas the survival of platelets from concentrates stored at 20° to 24°C is only about four days. Survival of platelets is affected by a variety of factors discussed below.

Factors affecting platelet recovery and survival after transfusion

1. *Compatibility* of platelets plays an important role in successful platelet therapy, because incompatible platelets may sensitise the recipient or may have a lower recovery and shorter survival in the presence of reactive antibodies in an already sensitised recipient.

ABO incompatibility

Patients requiring repeated blood transfusions should receive ABO compatible platelets. ABO incompatible platelets can be transfused when compatible platelets are not available, in an emergency, and when it is unlikely that repeated platelet transfusions will be required in the future. In patients who require HLA typed platelets, HLA matching takes precedence over ABO compatibility. Note that ABO incompatible platelet concentrates obtained by cell separator must have a low contamination with red cells.

Rhesus incompatibility has no effect on platelet recovery and survival, but transfusion of Rh(D)-positive platelets to a Rh(D)-negative recipient may result in sensitisation of the latter by contaminating red cells. For prevention of immunisation see p. 77.

HLA incompatibility is the main cause of immunisation to HLA antigens which gives rise to platelet 'refractoriness'. It is described in detail on p. 57.

Incompatibility due to platelet antigens is rarely the cause of poor recovery and shortened survival of platelets, except in the Pl^{A1}-negative recipient with anti-Pl^{A1} (p. 49).

2. *Spleen size.* Patients with splenomegaly may sequester and destroy in the spleen most of the transfused platelets.
3. *Infection, bleeding, DIC.* In the presence of any of these conditions, there will be little or no increment in the post-transfusion platelet count.
4. *Inappropriate storage of platelet concentrates.* Lack of agitation and inappropriate temperature of storage may result in a significant decrease in the expected recovery of platelets.

5. *Use of unsuitable filters* such as an in-line microaggregate filter, may cause a significant platelet loss. Similarly, carelessness in priming the administration set, or pooling of platelet concentrates may cause platelet losses.

Calculating the dose and post-transfusion increments

Dose of platelets

The required dose of platelets is calculated from body surface area, read off the nomogram using the patient's height and weight. A useful rule of thumb is that one unit of platelet concentrate, with at least 50×10^9 platelets, increases the platelet count one hour after transfusion by $10 \times 10^9/l$ per m² of body surface. The number of units of platelets required (n) can be calculated from the formula:

$$n = (P_1 - P_0) \times BSA/10$$

where P_1 and P_0 are the desired and initial platelet counts, respectively, and BSA is the patient's body surface area, estimated from the height and weight using the nomogram in Appendix II.

Example: how many units of platelets are required to raise the platelet count from $20 \times 10^9/l$ (P_0) to $60 \times 10^9/l$ (P_1) in a patient with body surface (BSA) of 1.5 m²?

$$n = (60 - 20) \times 1.5/10 = 6 \text{ units of platelets}$$

The formula does not take into account variations in the number of platelets in different units. Note that one unit of platelet concentrate harvested by apheresis is, for the purpose of calculating the dose, equivalent to five units of platelet concentrates obtained manually.

Post transfusion increment

The efficacy of platelet transfusion is estimated by calculating the platelet increment, related to the blood volume or body surface area. Many different formulae are in use for that purpose. One may simply write:

$$CI = (P_1 - P_0) \times BSA/n$$

where CI is the corrected increment of platelets, P_1 and P_0 are platelet counts determined one hour after and before transfusion, respectively, n is the number of units of platelets transfused, and BSA is the patient's body surface area (Appendix II). This method for the determination of the corrected increment of platelets does not take into account variation in the number of platelets in different units.

Example: a patient whose body surface (BSA) is 1.5 m² had a platelet count of $20 \times 10^9/l$ before (P_0) and $80 \times 10^9/l$ (P_1) one hour after receiving nine units of platelets (n); his corrected increment was:

$$CI = (80 - 20) \times 1.5/9 = 10 \times 10^9/l$$

Although the corrected increment is expressed as platelet count ($\times 10^9/l$) it is a relative figure which indicates the proportion of transfused platelets which remain in circulation one hour after transfusion. A CI higher than $7.5 \times 10^9/l$ would indicate a successful transfusion of platelets; CI of less than $7.5 \times 10^9/l$ indicates platelet refractoriness (see below). A CI estimated 24 hours after transfusion of platelets lower than $4.5 \times 10^9/l$, would indicate platelet refractoriness in the absence of any other condition which may affect both recovery and survival of platelets. Note that the results for platelet increments calculated using the above formula are not directly comparable to the results obtained using any other formula. No one method for calculating platelet increments has proven advantage over the others.

Procedures for transfusion

It is always best to use ABO and Rh group specific platelets. When these are not available use the ABO and Rh group-compatible platelets. ABO and Rh group-incompatible platelets can be used in an emergency, when compatible platelets are not available and when it is unlikely that the patient will require regular platelet transfusions in the future. Administer platelet concentrates through a platelet infusion set (p. 180); transfuse one pack at a time but there is no need to change the set between each pack. Alternatively, the standard administration set with a 170 μ filter may be used. The rate of transfusion depends on the circulatory state of the patient; in general platelets are given as quickly as possible. Recipients with a history of febrile or allergic reactions should be given an antihistamine (chlorpheniramine, Piriton, 10 mg) and hydrocortisone (100 mg) i.v. prior to transfusion.

INDICATIONS FOR PLATELET TRANSFUSION

---

1. Treatment or prevention of haemorrhage in bone marrow failure: aplastic anaemia, acute leukaemia and other haematological malignancies, as well as in patients with bone marrow suppression due to chemotherapy or irradiation.
2. Treatment of severe haemorrhage in, or preparation for surgery of, patients with qualitative disorders of platelets: Glanzmann's thrombasthenia, Bernard-Soulier syndrome, platelet storage pool disease, etc.
3. Treatment of severe bleeding after cardiopulmonary bypass, massive transfusion and exchange transfusion.
4. Possible indications for platelet transfusion:
   a. severe bleeding (CNS haemorrhage, massive gastrointestinal bleed) in immune thrombocytopenia (idiopathic thrombocytopenic purpura, drug induced thrombocytopenia, neonatal thrombocytopenia);
   b. life-threatening bleeding in thrombocytopenia caused by consumption of platelets as in disseminated intravascular coagulation, liver disease or hypersplenism.

*Remember that donor platelets will be removed from the
circulation as quickly as the recipient's platelets and that the
transfusion of platelets may prolong or aggravate the
underlying pathological process (DIC, ITP) and also cause
anaphylactoid reactions.*

5. Indication for use of HLA matched platelets is in sensitised
   patients with fully identified alloantibodies, requiring platelet
   support for a limited period of time, i.e. bone marrow
   transplantation, intensive chemotherapy and radiotherapy.

6. Indications for use of Pl^{A1}-negative platelets:
   a. Bleeding in patients with thrombasthenia who invariably
      lack the Pl^{A1} antigenic determinant. If transfused with
      random platelets they may produce anti-Pl^{A1} which will
      cause platelet refractoriness as well as febrile and
      anaphylactoid reactions.
   b. Bleeding in neonatal alloimmune purpura (p. 135).
   c. Bleeding in post-transfusion purpura (p. 146).

UNTOWARD EFFECTS AND PLATELET REFRACTORINESS

Alloimmunisation to platelet antigens and platelet refractoriness
Over two thirds of recipients of random donor platelet concentrates
become alloimmunised to HLA antigens and may develop refractoriness,
a term used to describe the failure of two consecutive platelet
transfusions to exceed the corrected increment of $7.5 \times 10^9/l$ determined
one hour after transfusion. Refractoriness does not usually occur during
the first two weeks of platelet transfusion. However, a proportion of
multiparous women, immunised during pregnancy, may display
refractoriness from the first platelet transfusion. In severely
immunosuppressed patients refractoriness may develop later but it may
have little effect on the recovery and survival of transfused platelets.

Patterns of alloimmunisation
There are two patterns of alloimmunisation:
1. restricted, in which alloantibodies are produced against one
   or two HLA antigens, usually A2, Bw4 or Bw6;
2. to multiple HLA antigens, and often to platelet antigens. In
   the first type of immunisation it is usually possible to provide
   HLA compatible platelets for transfusion, but in the second,
   the supply of compatible platelets can only be made possible
   if matched HLA siblings act as donors.

Investigation of platelet refractoriness
If refractoriness is suspected:
1. Check that the patient is afebrile, has no infection or
   splenomegaly and has a normal coagulation screen (no
   evidence of DIC).

2. Check that adequate number of platelet concentrates, stored at an appropriate temperature, are transfused using a correct administration set.
3. Check the patient's platelet count prior to and one hour after transfusion and calculate the corrected increment of platelets.
4. If corrected increment is less than $7.5 \times 10^9/l$ despite adequate numbers of platelets transfused, request laboratry tests for demonstrating alloantibodies. Lymphocytotoxicity tests are usually carried out for that purpose (p. 48).

Platelet administration in a 'refractory' patient
1. Identify the antibody(ies) and the pattern of alloimmunisation.
2. Provide, if possible, HLA matched platelets, i.e. negative for antigens A2, Bw4 or Bw6, collected by a blood cell processor. Such platelets should be ABO and Rh group compatible, and whenever possible, have a low content of leucocytes. Over 60% of HLA matched platelet transfusions are successful.
3. If the patient is refractory to HLA matched platelets, alloantibodies to other platelet antigens or multispecific HLA antibodies may have developed. Platelet cross-match, if available, should be carried out in an attempt to find compatible platelets (p. 49).
4. When platelet cross-match cannot be carried out or when no compatible units of platelets are found, the platelets given should be 'best match' from a single donor apheresed on a cell separator, since some haemostatic effect will be achieved despite refractoriness.

Febrile reactions, see p. 96.
Allergic reactions, see p. 99.
Granulocytopenia, see p. 98.
Transmission of infections, see p. 110.

REFERENCES

Kelton J G, Ali A M 1983 Platelet transfusion — a critical appraisal. In: Schiffer C A (ed) Transfusion support therapy. Clinics in Oncology 2: 549–585
Menitove J E 1983 Platelet transfusion for alloimmunised patients. In: Schiffer C A (ed) Transfusion support therapy. Clinics in Oncology 2: 587–609
Robinson E A E 1984 Single donor granulocytes and platelets. In: Bayer W L (ed) Blood transfusion and blood banking. Clinics in Haematology 13: 185–216

6. GRANULOCYTE TRANSFUSION

In recent years it has been realised that granulocyte transfusions are associated with potentially serious hazards and that this treatment should be reserved for a limited number of carefully selected cases where it is of proven benefit. These patients are almost invariably suffering from aplastic anaemia or acute leukaemia and are treated with intensive chemotherapy and/or irradiation during induction of remisssion or bone marrow transplantation.

PROPERTIES OF GRANULOCYTE CONCENTRATES

Methods of collection

Granulocyte concentrates can be prepared from single donations of blood or by leucapheresis. The two methods and their products are compared in Table 6.1.

Table 6.1 Characteristics of granulocyte concentrates

Characteristic	Method of collection	
	Manual (buffy coat)	Cell separator (leucapheresis)
Anticoagulant	ACD, CPD or CPDa-1	ACD(A) or ACD(B)
Sedimenting agent	none	dextran or HES*
Volume, ml	60	200 to 500
Granulocyte content, average, $\times\ 10^9$	0.6	10
Platelet content, average, $\times\ 10^9$	50	450
Red cell content, average, $\times\ 10^{12}$	0.18	0.60
Main potential risk	circulatory overload	pulmonary infiltration
Main advantage	none	suitable for HLA-typed concentrates
Cost	low	high

* HES, hydroxyethyl starch

Manual preparation is by harvesting the buffy coat layer, separated by centrifugation, from a single unit of blood. Each 'buffy coat' contains about 0.6×10^9 granulocytes, as well as many platelets and red cells suspended in a small volume of plasma. Buffy coats should be prepared within four hours, stored at 20°C and administered with 24 hours of blood collection.

Leucapheresis is the method of choice for preparation of granulocyte concentrates. Donors are healthy individuals usually given 6 mg of dexamethasone or 0.1 mg of etiocholanolone prior to leucapheresis for the purpose of increasing the circulating granulocyte count. Patients in the chronic phase of chronic granulocytic leukaemia can also serve as donors. Procedures used for leucapheresis are intermittent flow centrifugation (IFC) and continuous flow centrifugation (CFC) with or without dextran and hydroxyethyl starch (HES) used to sediment red cells quickly and thus increase the yield of granulocytes, filtration leucapheresis and gravity leucapheresis (p. 157). However, filtration leucapheresis cannot be recommended for use because activation of complement may take place during the procedure, and gravity leucapheresis is time consuming and labour intensive. Granulocyte concentrates are stored at 20°C and should be transfused without 24 hours of collection.

Dose of granulocytes and their recovery and survival

A transfusion of 10^{10} granulocytes a day is considered to be the effective dose. This is equivalent to 18 to 20 units of buffy coats or one unit of granulocyte concentrate collected by cell separator.

The recovery of granulocytes in the circulation is 50% one hour after transfusion in the first-time recipient and in the recipient of HLA-matched granulocytes. Recovery falls to 10% or even 5% in the presence of multispecific HLA antibodies in multiply-transfused patients. Granulocytes have a half life of seven to eight hours in the recipient's circulation.

Procedure for transfusion

Patients requiring a granulocyte transfusion for the first time should have ABO and Rh group specific granulocyte concentrates, daily, until their clinical condition improves. Patients who have received in the past multiple granulocyte transfusions, or blood transfusions, should receive whenever possible granulocyte concentrates donated by HLA matched or partially matched donors.

Prior to transfusion red cells compatibility testing must be carried out, as granulocyte concentrates contain large numbers of red cells.

The recipient of granulocyte concentrates is usually given prophylactic hydrocortisone, 100 mg, and an antihistamine such as chlorpheniramine (Piriton) 10 mg, both i.v. The granulocyte concentrates are administered using a blood administration set at a rate not exceeding 5×10^9 granulocytes per square metre of body surface per hour. In practice this means, for an adult, transfusing ten buffy coats in an hour, and a unit of granulocyte concentrate obtained using a cell separator in two hours.

INDICATIONS FOR GRANULOCYTE TRANSFUSION

1. Neutropenic patients who satisfy the following criteria:
   a. granulocyte count less than $0.2 \times 10^9/l$, and neutropenia *not* on the point of recovery, as judged by the therapeutic regimens used or bone marrow aspirate;
   b. clear evidence of bacterial infection: bacteriological cultures positive or clinical evidence e.g. lobar infiltrate on chest X-ray, skin abscess, etc;
   c. good evidence that antibiotics have failed after 48–72 hours of treatment: e.g. persistent fever and signs of progressive infection (positive cultures, expanding pulmonary or skin lesions, septicaemic shock). The presence of high fever without other evidence of bacterial infection may indicate a viral or fungal infection in which the use of granulocyte concentrates is of unproven value.
2. The benefit of granulocyte concentrates in neonates with severe neutropenia and septicaemia has been reported (Laurenti et al, 1978) but the value of the treatment has not yet been established.
   Note that prophylactic use of granulocyte concentrates is not justified as the hazards of treatment outweigh the doubtful benefits.

UNTOWARD EFFECTS OF GRANULOCYTE TRANSFUSION

1. **Febrile reactions** are common, immediate and may be very severe. The incidence of febrile reactions is high, and almost every recipient of repeated granulocyte transfusions experiences at least one episode of fever. The mechanisms responsible for pyrexia are complex and include reaction between granulocyte and HLA antigens and corresponding antibodies, and the effect of inflammatory mediators released from granulocytes damaged during the preparation of the concentrate. Administration of aspirin, 300 mg orally, prior to transfusion may be helpful, but rarely abolishes the fever entirely (p. 96).
2. **Pulmonary infiltration** is the most serious hazard of granulocyte transfusions. Pulmonary infiltrates are common in severely neutropenic patients with acute myeloid leukaemia whether or not they receive granulocyte transfusions. However, the incidence of pulmonary infiltrates is increased twofold in patients receiving granulocyte transfusions. The mechanism responsible is complex and involves fluid overload, pulmonary oedema, antibody mediated sequestration of granulocytes in the lungs and infection. The mortality associated with pulmonary infiltrates occurring with granulocyte transfusions is about 35%.

Clinical manifestations

In the most severe cases acute respiratory distress develops during or within minutes of completion of a granulocyte transfusion. The chest X-ray reveals diffuse infiltration of both lungs. In the less severe cases signs and symtoms similar to those in lobar pneumonia develop within hours of transfusion. The mild form of pulmonary infiltrates is asymptomatic but the infiltrates can be seen on chest X-ray.

Management

If the patient becomes breathless, begins to cough or complains of chest pain, granulocyte transfusion must be discontinued immediately. Chest X-ray is carried out and if infiltrates are present arterial blood gases are determined. Severely affected patients are best treated in an intensive care unit with respiratory, cardiovascular, renal and nutritional support. Artificial ventilation is usually required. It is important to deal with pulmonary oedema, circulatory overload and hyperviscosity syndrome at the same time (see below). The less severely affected patients do not require management in the intensive care unit, but circulatory overload and hyper-viscosity must always be treated since they may aggravate the lung lesion.

Granulocyte transfusions should *never* be given to patients receiving systemic amphotericin B, because in these patients pulmonary infiltrates occur with high frequency and in a severe form.

3. **Circulatory overload and hyperviscosity syndrome.** Granulocyte concentrates contain many red cells (Table 6.1) and when administered to patients without anaemia they may cause an unacceptable increase in haemoglobin concentration and PCV; for buffy coats, each unit raises the haemoglobin concentration by approximately 0.1 g/dl. Venesection may be required in some patients to reduce the PCV. By the same token, transfusion of blood or red cells should be avoided during the period of treatment with granulocyte concentrates, unless the haemoglobin concentration is very low.

4. **Alloimmunisation to granulocyte antigens.** The majority of patients receiving granulocyte transfusions develop HLA and granulocyte antibodies with all the associated problems such as platelet refractoriness (p. 57) and likelihood of febrile reactions (see above).

5. **Transmission of infection** (p. 110).

6. **Graft versus host disease** (p. 97).

REFERENCES

Laurenti F, La Greca G, Ferro R, Bucci G 1978 Transfusions of polymorphonuclear neutrophils in a premature infant with Klebsiella sepsis. Lancet 2: 111–112
Robinson E A E 1984 Single donor granulocytes and platelets. In: Bayer W L (ed) Blood Transfusion and blood banking. Clinics in Haematology 13: 185–216
Strauss R G 1983 Granulocyte transfusion therapy. In: Schiffer C (ed) Transfusion support therapy. Clinics in Oncology 2: 635–655

7. TRANSFUSION OF PLASMA COMPONENTS AND PRODUCTS

Plasma components, fresh frozen plasma and cryoprecipitate, are prepared by simple mechanical separation of cells from plasma* using centrifugation and by freezing. Plasma components contain most of the plasma constituents including the anticoagulant used. *Plasma products* are produced by fractionation and purification of specific proteins, e.g. albumin, coagulation factors and immunoglobulins. The main advantages and disadvantages of plasma components and products are listed in Table 7.1.

Table 7.1 Advantages and disadvantages of single unit and small pool plasma components and of products fractionated from pooled plasma

Preparation	Advantages	Disadvantages
Single unit and small pool components, frozen	instant availability ease and speed of preparation low cost of preparation	variation in potency of active factors storage temperature below −30°C
	low rate of disease transmission to the recipient	inconvenient administration — thawing and large volume of preparation allergic reactions presence of undesirable active and inert constituents short shelf life
Products fractionated from pooled plasma, freeze dried	specified potency	require technology for collection and fractionation of plasma
	ease of administration — no preparation and small volume of product storage at 4°C greatly reduced incidence of allergic reactions greatly reduced content of undesirable active and inert substances long shelf life	potentially high rate of disease transmission to the recipient high cost of preparation

FRESH FROZEN PLASMA

Definition
Fresh frozen plasma (FFP) for clinical use is separated from single units of blood and rapidly frozen within six hours after donation.

* In this Chapter 'plasma' is used to denote 'human plasma'.

Properties
FFP is ABO and Rh group specific. The volume of one unit of FFP
prepared from a single donation is approximately 200 ml. Units of plasma
collected by machine plasmapheresis may have up to 500 ml and packs of
PPF for paediatric use contain 50 to 100 ml.

Storage and shelf-life
FFP, kept in a deep-freeze at a temperature below –30°C has a shelf-life
of one year. When FFP is kept at –20°C its shelf-life is shorter, and the
inventory control should ensure its rapid turnover.

Administration
FFP should be thawed in a 37°C water bath with a stirrer, with frequent
agitation by hand. It should never be thawed under the hot water tap. It
should be administered within half an hour after thawing as the activity
of coagulation factors V and VIII is rapidly lost on standing. FFP is given
intravenously through a blood administration set with a filter, at a flow
rate not greater than 10 ml/min.

Indications for use

1. Treatment of congenital deficiencies of factors V and XI.
2. Replacement of coagulation factors in the following diseases
   and disorders: DIC, liver disease, deficiency of vitamin K
   dependent coagulation factors, overdose of oral
   anticoagulants, massive transfusion of stored blood, during
   cardio-pulmonary bypass, and in multiple large volume
   plasma exchanges.
3. Urgent replacement of missing haemostatic factors, when
   specific concentrate preparations are not immediately
   available: haemophilia A, haemophilia B, deficiency of factors
   VII, X and prothrombin, von Willebrand's disease, deficiency
   of factors XIII and fibrinogen, and antithrombin III
   deficiency.
4. In conditions in which it is expected that one of the following
   plasma constituents is lacking: (a) fibronectin in septicaemia
   and in failure of wound healing; (b) PGI_2-inducing activity in
   thrombotic thrombocytopenic purpura; (c) C_1 esterase
   inhibitor in hereditary angio-neurotic oedema.
5. For resuspension of group O red cells for transfusion to
   infants with ABO haemolytic disease of the newborn
   (p. 134); as a rule group AB plasma is used.
6. For transfusion to patients with anti-Le[a] and/or anti-Le[b]
   antibodies prior to transfusion with Le(a+b+) blood when
   Le(a–b–) blood is not available. For this purpose FFP should
   be donated by donors who are known secretors (possessing
   the *Se* gene).

Volume and frequency of administration depend on clinical indications
which should be assessed for each patient separately. In practice, two to
five units of FFP (5 to 15 ml/kg body weight) are administered to the

patient with a congenital deficiency of one of the haemostatic factors; two to four units, or as much as may be tolerated without overloading the circulation, is administered daily to patients with one of the conditions or diseases listed under (2) and (4) above, although the dose of or even the need for FFP in the latter group has not been generally agreed on. In thrombotic thrombocytopenic purpura daily administration may be required for long periods of time.

Untoward effects and contraindications

1. Urticaria and anaphylactoid reactions; avoid administration to individuals with a history of bonchial asthma, urticaria or previous severe reaction to plasma (p. 99).
2. Circulatory overload (p. 102).
3. Non-haemolytic febrile transfusion reaction (p. 96).
4. Reaction caused by vasoactive substances (p. 105).
5. Transmission of diseases (p. 110).

CRYOPRECIPITATE

Definition.
A plasma component containing factor VIII and fibrinogen, obtained from a single donation of fresh plasma by rapid freezing within six hours of collection, subsequent thawing at 4 to 8°C, and removal of supernatant.

Properties
Cryoprecipitate is ABO and Rh group specific. The volume of one unit is on average 20 ml, and contains about 80 i.u. of factor VIII:C (the i.u. is defined by the activity of the international reference preparation), similar amount of VIII:vW, about 0.25 g of fibrinogen, as well as half of the amount of factor XIII and fibronectin present in the original donation. Recovery in the patient of infused factor VIII:C is over 80% and its plasma half-life about 12 hours. The recovery of factor VIII:RAg is similar, but its half-life is longer, about 24 hours. Freeze-dried cryoprecipitate in single units or small pools (pooled from six to 12 single units) are prepared by a number of Blood Transfusion Centres.

Storage and shelf-life
Cryoprecipitate is stable for up to one year when kept at a temperature below −30°C.

Administration
Thaw rapidly the required number of packs of cryoprecipitate at 37°C in water bath with manual agitation, remove the packs as soon as thawed and pool their content into a large syringe or transfer pack. Rinse each pack with a small volume of sterile saline (usually 10 to 20 ml) and add it to the pool. Administer as soon as possible, and not later than one hour after thawing, preferably using a component administration set, at a rate not exceeding 10 ml per minute.

Indications for use

1. Treatment or prevention of bleeding in haemophilia A and von Willebrand's disease.
2. The corresponding treatment of congenital factor XIII deficiency, afibrinogenaemia and disfibrinogenaemia.
3. Rarely, for correcting factor VIII deficiency induced by massive transfusion.
4. In treatment of intractable bleeding in uraemia and some platelet function disorders (Hermansky-Pudlak syndrome, platelet storage pool disease, etc.).

The dose of factor VIII for treatment of haemophilia A and von Willebrand's disease is calculated using the formula:

$$D = BW \times I/2$$

where D is the dose in i.u., BW body weight in kg, and I the desired increment in i.u./dl. A unit of cryoprecipitate contains on average 80 i.u. of factor VIII. Varying degrees of severity of bleeding in haemophilia A require different concentrations of factor VIII:C and the requirements can be worked out from Table 7.2. Whenever possible the response to treatment should be assessed by plasma factor VIII:C assays; major surgery should not be undertaken if this cannot be done. In von Willebrand's disease there is a characteristic late rise in the plasma concentration of factor VIII:C after cryoprecipitate infusion. The initial treatment is as for haemophilia but the frequency of infusions is determined by assaying factor VIII:C. For further details, specialised literature should be consulted (see references).

Table 7.2 Dose of factor VIII:C for different situations in haemophilia A

Situation	Required plasma conc. i.u./dl	Initial dose of factor VIII, i.u./kg b.w.	Number of infusions required, and interval of administration
Minor spontaneous haemarthroses and haematomata	15–20	8–10	1–3 times, 24 hourly
Severe haemarthroses, muscle haematomata, minor surgery	20–40	10–20	3–7 times, 12 hourly initially, then 24 hourly
Major surgery,* CNS bleeding	80–100	40–50	12 hourly, until normal healing and rehabilitation completed

* Major surgery in haemophilia should only be undertaken in special centres experienced in its haematological management.

Untoward effects

1. Urticaria and anaphylactoid reactions (p. 99).
2. Circulatory overload (p. 102).
3. Reaction caused by vasoactive substances (p. 105).
4. Bleeding tendency due to very high fibrinogen concentration achieved after infusion of a large number of cryoprecipitate units.
5. Transmission of diseases (p. 110).

FACTOR VIII CONCENTRATE

Definition
A freeze-dried (lyophilised) preparation of factor VIII obtained by
fractionation from large pools of fresh frozen plasma.

Properties
Factor VIII concentrate is a white or yellowish powder in a vial,
packaged with sterile water for reconstitution. The registered name,
activity of factor VIII:C, other constituents, instructions for reconstitution
and expiry date are stated on the label (as well as other information
required by the licensing authority) and must be checked before
administration. Different preparations may differ in their content of
factor VIII:C, but vials usually contain 250, 500 or 1000 i.u. *Intermediate
purity* concentrates usually have 15 i.u. of factor VIII:C per millilitre of
reconstituted preparation, whereas *high purity* concentrates contain 20 to
30 i.u./ml. Group specific concentrates are available for patients with
blood group A or B, and also concentrates rendered free from the risk of
virus transmission by an additional heat-sterilisation process. Most factor
VIII concentrates also contain:
   1. Factor VIII:vW in varying amounts, less of it and in an
      altered molecular form in the high purity concentrates. These
      concentrates should not be used for treatment of von
      Willebrand's disease.
   2. Fibrinogen in varying amounts, but less in the high purity
      concentrates.
   3. Naturally occurring anti-A and anti-B agglutinins.
   4. Heparin, about 1 i.u./ml.
   5. Traces of other plasma proteins.
   6. Stabilising agents, such as dextrose.

Storage and shelf-life
Factor VIII concentrate is stored at 6 to 8°C and has a shelf-life of up to
two years. Some preparations can be kept at room temperature for up to
six months.

Administration
The dose is calculated as described for cryoprecipitate (p. 66). Warm
the vials to room temperature. Add sterile water, according to
instructions, through a wide bore needle (a special double lumen needle
is provided by some manufacturers.). Swirl gently to avoid frothing.
When the powder is completely dissolved draw the solution into a syringe
or administration set and administer intravenously through a needle,
butterfly or venflow at a rate not exceeding 2 ml/min. Administer within
one hour of reconstitution. Do not refrigerate reconstituted material.
Discard the material if a gel forms at any time.

Indications for use
   1. Treatment or prevention of bleeding in patients with
      haemophilia A.

2. Treatment of bleeding in patients with severe von Willebrand's disease; note that only intermediate purity concentrates should be used.
3. Treatment of bleeding in patients with factor VIII:C antibodies.

The dose of factor VIII:C required is calculated using Table 7.2 and the formula on p. 66. For prophylactic treatment 250 to 1000 i.u. of factor VIII:C are administered two to three times weekly. Patients with antibodies to factor VIII:C require very large doses of concentrate, administered two to six times dailly by injection or by continuous infusion until the antibody is no longer detectable. Within five to seven days of starting therapy, the antibody titre rises to a very high level and factor VIII concentrates are no longer effective. Simultaneously to treatment with factor VIII concentrate plasma exchange may be used to 'wash out' the antibody. Alternatively, patients with factor VIII antibody may be treated with porcine factor VIII or with factor IX concentrates (p. 69).

The patient's response should be monitored with factor VIII:C assay. Failure to achieve a rise of factor VIII:C concentration in the plasma may be due to: wrongly calculated dose, severe bleeding (loss of factor VIII:C) or development of antibodies. In addition, there are individual variations of the recovery of factor VIII:C in the plasma and its half-life, which are particularly obvious with high purity factor VIII concentrates.

Untoward effects

1. Urticaria and anaphylactoid reactions (p. 99).
2. Non-haemolytic febrile transfusion reactions (p. 96).
3. Reaction caused by vasoactive substances (p. 105).
4. Development of antibodies to factor VIII.
5. Haemolysis due to the presence of isoagglutinins. This occurs only when large doses of factor VIII concentrate are administered frequently to patients with antibodies to factor VIII. Monitor recipients who are blood group A, B or AB for a fall in the haemoglobin concentration, haemoglobinaemia or a rising reticulocyte count. Transfuse if necessary with group O blood or packed cells. Thereafter use group specific factor VIII concentrate.
6. Transmission of diseases (p. 110).

FACTOR IX CONCENTRATE

Definition
A freeze-dried preparation of factors IX, X and prothrombin prepared by fractionation from large pools of plasma.

Properties
Factor IX concentrate is a white or yellowish powder in a vial. When reconstituted according to instructions, it contains 30 to 100 i.u. of factor

IX and the same number of units of factor X and prothrombin per ml of solution. Some preparations also contain factor VII in concentration of 25 to 30 u/ml. Certain preparations of factor IX concentrate, Feiba (Immuno) and Autoplex (Hyland), contain partially activated factors IX, X and prothrombin, and are used solely for the therapy of bleeding episodes in patients with factor VIII antibodies. Specific factor VII concentrates are also available.

Storage and shelf-life

Factor IX concentrate are stable at 6 to 8°C for up to two years.

Administration

Dissolve the concentrate with sterile water according to instructions. Swirl the solution gently to avoid frothing. Administer as soon as possible, but not later than three hours after reconstitution, using a syringe or a transfer pack, through a needle, butterfly or venflow. The rate of infusion should not exceed 2 ml/min.

Indications for use

1. Treatment or prevention of bleeding in factor IX deficiency (haemophilia B, Christmas disease).
2. Treatment or prevention of bleeding in factor VII, X and prothrombin deficiency and defects.
3. Treatment of life-threatening bleeding caused by an overdose of oral anticoagulants, when the patient is unable to tolerate the necessary volume of fresh frozen plasma.
4. Treatment of bleeding in patients with factor VIII antibodies. Both activated and conventional preparations can be used, but the activated preparations are more effective in arresting bleeding.

Dose

The plasma concentration of factor IX required to arrest different types of bleeding is shown on Table 7.3. The recovery of factor IX is about 50% and its plasma half-life 18 to 36 hours. Whenever possible, the response to infusion should be monitored by factor IX assays.

The dose of factor IX concentrate used for treating other congenital

Table 7.3 Dose of factor IX for different situations in haemophilia B (Christmas disease)

Situation	Required plasma conc. i.u./dl*	Initial dose in i.u./kg body weight	Number of infusions required and interval of administration
Prophylaxis	5	40–60	once per week
Minor spontaneous haemarthroses and haematomata	5–15	15	1–3 infusions 24 hourly
Severe haemarthrosis	15–30	20–30	2–5 infusions 24 hourly
Major surgery**	over 50	50–75	12 or 24 hourly until healing and mobilisation completed

* 1 i.u. of factor IX per kg body weight generally increase factor IX concentration in plasma by 1 i.u./dl.

** Major surgery in haemophilia should only be undertaken in special centres experienced in its haematological management.

Table 7.4 Haemostatic levels, dose and plasma half-life of factors X, VII and prothrombin

Factor	Haemostatic level in plasma %	Usual initial dose u/kg b.w.	Plasma half-life, hours
X	10–20	15	40–50
VII	5–10	10	4–6
Prothrombin	40	20	70–80

deficiencies is shown on Table 7.4. Patients bleeding after an overdose of oral anticoagulants are usually given a single dose of 5 to 10 u/kg body weight.

Patients with antibodies to factor VIII:C who are bleeding are given 60 to 100 u of an activated preparation of factor IX per kg body weight at eight to 12 h intervals. This is repeated until there is clinical improvement. The effective dose depends on the severity of bleeding and doses as high as 150 u/kg body weight have been given hourly. Factor VIII concentrate is administered after each dose. Note that the potency of activated preparations is defined by manufacturers on the basis of its ability to shorten the clotting times of plasma with high titre antibody.

Untoward effects

1. Thrombogenicity. Factor IX concentrates accelerate coagulation and have been implicated in DIC and thrombotic episodes. These risks are particularly dangerous with activated preparations; the platelet count and the FDP concentration must be determined serially and infusion stopped if the count falls below $60 \times 10^9/l$ or if the FDP in the plasma rises above 20 μg/ml.
   Note that factor IX concentrates are contraindicated in DIC, liver disease and in the neonate.
2. Flushing, headache and tingling due to the presence of vasoactive substances.
3. Urticaria and anaphylactoid reactions (p. 99).
4. Development of an antibody in a patient with a congenital deficiency of factor IX.
5. Transmission of diseases (p. 110).

FIBRINOGEN CONCENTRATE

Definition
A freeze dried preparation of fibrinogen produced by fractionation from small pools of plasma.

Properties
White or yellowish powder in a vial, each containing 1 or 2 g of fibrinogen. It may be stored in the dark at room temperature for up to two years.

Administration
Reconstitute with sterile water according to instructions. Swirl gently to

avoid frothing. When completely dissolved, administer slowly, no longer than three hours after reconstitution, always using an administration set with a filter.

Indications for use

Fibrinogen concentrate is not recommended for use in the U.K. and cryoprecipitate should be used instead for treatment of bleeding in congenital fibrinogen deficiency and dysfibrinogenaemia.

Note that fibrinogen concentrate should not be administered in DIC and/or liver disease, as it may aggravate the thrombotic tendency.

Topical use of fibrinogen concentrate for arresting bleeding should be discouraged; fibrinogen solution tends to be washed away by the flowing blood.

Dose

The minumum concentration of fibrinogen in the plasma required for sustained haemostasis is between 0.05 and 0.1 g/l. Its half life is about 90 hours. The initial dose is 2 to 4 g, repeated in three to four days, if required.

Untoward effects

    1. Thromboembolism.

    2. Risk of transmitting hepatitis.

OTHER CONCENTRATES OF COAGULATION FACTORS

Factor XIII and *factor XI concentrates* were used in the past but the safety and availability of cryoprecipitate and fresh frozen plasma have made the concentrates obsolete.

Antithrombin III concentrates (Kabi; Behringwerke) are used for treating thrombotic episodes in patients with congenital antithrombin III deficiency. The suggested dose is 50 units/kg body weight, to achieve a plasma concentration of 80% or higher. The infusion (usually 30 u/kg body weight) is repeated at 12 or 24 hour intervals, depending on the results obtained by assaying antithrombin III. No untoward effects of antithrombin III were noted in a small group of patients treated.

ALBUMIN PREPARATIONS

Definition

Protein solutions containing predominantly albumin prepared by fractionation of large pools of plasma.

Properties

There are two types of albumin preparations available, plasma protein fraction (PPF) and albumin solution, the latter having a greater degree of purity. In the U.K. both preparations, available from the Blood Products

Laboratory, Elstree, have high purity (over 95%) and they differ only in the protein concentration which is 5% and 20%, respectively, and content of salts which is four times lower in the albumin solution.

1. *PPF* is a pale yellow or brown, clear solution of proteins, 5 g/dl, of which over 90% is albumin. The remaining proteins are alpha- and beta-globulins. The solution contains less than 2 mmol/l of potassium, 15 mmol/l of citrate and 160 mmol/l of sodium. Different stabilisers are added by fractionators to their products. PPF may be stored in the dark, at room temperature, for up to five years. PPF, supplied by the Blood Products Laboratory, Elstree, to the NHS, comes in 100 ml and 400 ml bottles, but commercially available PPF comes in 50 ml, 100 ml, 200 ml and 500 ml bottles.

2. *Salt poor albumin* is a pale yellow or brown solution of albumin 20 g/l. It contains less than 10 mmol/l of potassium, 20 mmol/l of citrate and 130 mmol/l of sodium. It comes in 100 ml bottles.

Administration

PPF and albumin are ready for administration. In some countries, however, freeze-dried albumin is also available and it must be reconstituted according to instructions. Discard bottles which are cloudy. Administer using an infusion set with a filter, at a rate not exceeding 16 ml/min, though a higher rate of infusion can be used if the CVP is monitored.

Indications for use and dosage

The indication for use of PPF (5% albumin solution) is the replacement of plasma proteins and expansion of plasma volume as in:

1. Hypoproteinaemia following burns, and occaisonally, extensive surgery. In these conditions 500 to 2000 ml of PPF are administered initially followed by adequate volumes of PPF to maintain the concentration of plasma albumin between 25 and 30 g/l. The recommended dose for children is 20 to 30 ml per kg body weight.

2. As the replacement fluid in plasma-exchange, and sometimes for priming the pump in cardiopulmonary bypass.

3. Haemorrhagic shock; but note that crystalloid solutions are as effective as PPF while awaiting blood (p. 83).

The indication for use of 20% albumin solution is solely the replacement of plasma proteins as in:

1. Severe hypoproteinaemia in acute nephrotic syndrome and acute liver disease. Adults should receive 100 to 400 ml daily, and children 1.5 to 6 ml/kg body weight in 24 hours. Diuretics are essential when oedema is present, because every 10 ml of 20% albumin pulls 35 ml of extravascular fluid into the circulation within 15 min of administration.

2. Hyperbilirubinaemia in the newborn when 5 to 10 ml of salt-

poor albumin may be added to the blood used for exchange transfusion.

3. Toxaemia of pregnancy when the daily administration of 50 ml of salt poor albumin may be beneficial.
4. In some cases of Gram-negative septicaemia.

Albumin preparations are not indicated for the treatment of hypoproteinaemia in malnutrition, chronic nephrotic syndrome or cirrhosis.

Note that albumin preparations contain no coagulation factors and cannot be used to correct a haemostatic defect.

Untoward effects

1. Urticaria and anaphylactoid reactions (p. 99).
2. Febrile reactions (p. 96).
3. Circulatory overload is a particular risk: always watch carefully for pulmonary oedema (p. 102).
4. Hypotension due to the presence of vasoactive substances from plasma. This effect is seen only in some batches of PPF when the rate of administration exceeds 10 ml/min.

NORMAL AND SPECIFIC IMMUNOGLOBULINS

Definition

Normal immunoglobulin is a preparation obtained by fractionation of plasma collected from selected donors or from human placentae.

Specific immunoglobulins are preparations obtained by fractionation of plasma from donors who possess a high titre of specific antibodies in the plasma.

Properties

Immunoglobulin preparations are pale brown or yellow, clear solutions, or when freeze-dried yield a whitish powder. *Normal immunoglubulin*, for intramuscular injection, contains a mixture of immunoglobulins present in the healthy adult population: antibodies against poliomyelitis, measles and diphtheria, as well as against hepatitis A and non-A, non-B hepatitis. It is available in vials containing 250 mg and 750 mg of protein.

Normal immunoglobulin, for intravenous administration, is specially prepared immunoglobulin preparation, free from aggregated forms, with preserved Fc receptor site, and devoid of side effects.

Specific immunoglobulins, for intramuscular injection, are prepared from plasma containing a high titre of antibodies against a specific pathogen. Specific immunoglobulins available in the U.K. are listed in Table 7.5. Anti-D immunoglobulin is described in detail on p. 76. Other specific immunoglobulins, for example anti-pseudomonas aeruginosa immunoglobulin, may be available in some countries.

Table 7.5 Uses of human immunoglobulins in the prevention and treatment of viral and bacterial infections

Condition	Population requiring IG	Preparation*	Dose
Hepatitis A	family contacts institutional outbreaks	IG	3.2 mg/kg body wt.
	travellers to endemic areas	IG	3.2 mg/kg body wt.
Hepatitis non A, non B,	percutaneous or mucosal exposure	IG	8 mg/kg body wt.
Hepatitis B	percutaneous or mucosal exposure	HBIG	8–11 mg/kg body wt. repeated in 1 month
	newborns of mothers with HBsAg	HBIG	8 mg at birth, at 3 and 6 months
	sexual contacts of acute Hep. B patients	HBIG	8 mg/kg body wt., Repeated at 1 month
Rubella	women exposed during early pregnancy	IG	20 ml
Varicella-zoster	immunosuppressed contacts or newborn contacts	VZIG	12–15 units/kg body wt. minimum 125 μ
Measles	infants less than 1 year old or immunosuppressed contact if exposure less than 6 days previously	IG	0.25 ml/kg body wt. or 0.5 ml/kg body wt. if immunosuppressed
Rabies	subjects exposed to rabid animals	RIG	20 iu/kg body wt.
Tetanus	following significant exposure of non immunised or incompletely immunised person; immediately on diagnosis of disease	TIG	250 units for prophylaxis 3000–6000 units for therapy

Modified from Bull. World Health Org. 1982
* IG, normal immunoglobulin; HBIG, anti-HBs immunoglobulin; VZIG, anti-varicella-zoster immunoglobulin; RIG, anti-rabies immunoglobulin; TIG, anti-tetanus immunoglobulin.

Storage and shelf-life

Immunoglobulin preparations are stable when kept at 4 to 6°C for up to two years.

Administration

No preparation is required for immunoglobulins in solution; freeze-dried preparations are reconstituted according to the manufacturers' instructions. Preparations for intramuscular injection are administered deeply into the muscle, and those for intravenous injection are administered slowly.

Indications for use and dosage

1. Prevention and treatment of diseases responsive to administration of normal or specific immunoglobulins. The list of diseases, population requiring it, type of preparation and dosage are given in Table 7.5. All immunoglobulins are administered intramuscularly, with the exception of the high dose antitetanus immunoglobulin preparation for intravenous injection, reserved for administration at the onset of the disease. In England and Wales immunoglobulin preparations

are available on application to laboratories of the Public Health Laboratory Service, who also provide advice on their use.

2. Replacement therapy with normal immunoglobulin in patients with antibody deficiency syndromes resulting from defective antibody synthesis whether congenital or acquired. The initial loading dose is 200 to 500 mg/kg body weight, aimed to raise serum IgG levels to over 2 g/l. To reduce discomfort the immunoglobulin is injected in divided doses over a period of week. It is followed by injections of at least 25 mg/kg body weight at one, two, three or four week intervals, to maintain the initial increase. If symptoms and signs of antibody deficiency are not controlled, larger doses to achieve immunoglobulin levels of up to 10 g/l may be required. Conditions and diseases in which normal immunoglobulin can be used are listed in Table 7.6.

3. Treatment of immune haematological disease (idiopathic thrombocytopenic purpura (ITP), particularly in children and immune neutropenia). Recent reports have indicated that in children, and to a lesser extent in adults, the intravenous administration of high dose immunoglobulin can provoke a predictable rise in platelet count lasting for days, weeks or even months. The recommended dose is 400 mg/kg body weight daily for five days. The platelet count rises within five to ten days of starting therapy. When the platelet count falls or bleeding recurs repeated infusions can be given.

Table 7.6 Conditions where replacement therapy with normal immunoglobulin may be justified

X-linked agammaglobulinaemia
Varied immunodeficiency
Ig deficiency with raised IgM,
Immunodeficiency with thymoma
Severe combined immunodeficiency
Any patient lacking IgM
Ataxia telangiectasia
Wiskott-Aldrich syndrome
Thymic hypoplasia
Drug induced T cell defects
? chronic lymphatic leukaemia
? multiple myeloma

Untoward effects

1. Systemic effects are
   a. early, anaphylactic reaction
   b. late, urticaria, arthralgia, rash and diarrhoea.
2. Local effects are pain, inflammation and induration at the site of injection.

Reactions to immunoglobulin may be troublesome in patients receiving long term replacement therapy. Systemic reactions may be prevented or minimised by an injection of hydrocortisone (100 mg i.v.) prior to administration and/or by oral aspirin or antihistamines before and for two to six days following the injection. Local reactions are prevented by injecting smaller volumes of immunoglobulin either as a divided dose or at shorter intervals, using multiple sites.

ANTI-D IMMUNOGLOBULIN

Definition
Anti-D(Rh_o) immunoglobulin is a preparation of incomplete antibodies to D antigen of human red blood cells.

Properties
It is obtained by fractionation from pooled plasma from donors naturally or deliberately immunised to D antigen. It is a solution containing anti-D, small amounts of anti-C, anti-E and anti-c antibodies. Vials containing 50 μg (250 i.u.), 100 μg (500 i.u.) and 500 μg (2500 i.u.) for intramuscular injection and at least 100 μg (500 i.u.) for intravenous injection, are available on request from the Regional Transfusion Centres in England and Wales, and from national fractionators or commercial sources in other countries.

Storage and shelf-life
Anti-D immunoglobulin is stable in the dark for up to two years when stored at 2 to 8°C.

Administration
No preparation is necessary. Anti-D immunoglobulin is administered by deep intramuscular injection. Only preparations intended for intravenous administration can be given by infusion.

Indications for use and dosage
1. Prevention of sensitisation in Rh(D) negative women to fetal Rh(D) positive red cells during pregnancy or at birth.
   a. Following delivery, Rh(D)-negative women giving birth to a Rh(D)-positive infant should receive 100 μg (500 i.u.) of anti-D immunoglobulin by deep intramuscular injection not later than 72 hours after delivery*. It is advisable to perform the Kleihauer test on a sample of mother's blood (p. 78), and if more than 4 ml of fetal red cells are detected in the circulation, an additional 25 μg (125 i.u.) should be given for each millilitre of fetal cells. The management of massive transplacental haemorrhage is essentially the same as that following inadvertent transfusion of Rh(D)-positive red cells (see below).
   b. Following amniocentesis, external version or antepartum haemorrhage in Rh(D)-negative pregnant women, 100 μg

---

* In some countries the recommended dose is 200 or even 300 μg (1000 or 1500 i.u.).

(500 i.u.) of anti-D immunoglobulin should be given by deep intramuscular injection within 48 hours.

c. Following miscarriage or termination of pregnancy in Rh(D)-negative women, 50 µg (250 i.u.) of anti-D immunoglobulin should be given in a pregnancy of less than 20 weeks and 100 µg (500 i.u.) thereafter, by deep intramuscular injection within 48 hours.

Although there is evidence that administration of anti-D immunoglobulin during uncomplicated pregnancy, as an antenatal prophylaxis for all Rh(D)-negative women, may reduce the incidence of Rh sensitisation, the procedure has not yet been introduced for routine use in the U.K.

2. Prevention of sensitisation of Rh(D)-negative women of the reproductive age following transfusion of Rh(D)-positive blood and blood components.

a. Intramuscular route: A single dose of 25 µg (125 i.u.) per each ml of Rh(D)-positive red cells which the patient had received, is given. When a large volume must be given, the dose is divided.

b. Intravenous route: 10 to 15 µg (50 to 75 i.u.) of the intravenous preparation per ml of Rh(D)-positive red cells is administered as a slow infusion, not exceeding a total of 2500 µg in a single dose. The infusion may be repeated 12 hourly until the desired total dose of anti-D immunoglobulin is administered.

For prevention of sensitisation of Rh(D)-negative women by transfusion of Rh(D)-positive platelets, which contain small numbers of red cells, it is sufficient to give 100 µg (500 i.u.) of anti-D immunoglobulin, intramuscularly, for every six to eight units of single platelet concentrates, or one to two units of platelet concentrates obtained by platelet apheresis.

Management of inadvertent transfusion of Rh(D)-positive red cells or a large transplacental haemorrhage (TPH) in a Rh(D) negative woman of reproductive age

The decision whether to attempt to prevent sensitisation of a Rh(D)-negative woman of reproductive age following inadvertent transfusion of Rh(D)-positive red cells or transplacental haemorrhage (TPH) is made after assessment of each case, as follows:

1. Determine the volume of Rh(D)-positive red cells in the circulation. Following transfusion the volume of red cells can be estimated from the number of units of blood administered. In TPH Kleihauer's test must be used for calculating the size of the TPH.

2. Calculate the required dose of anti-D immunoglobulin and decide whether the preparation for intramuscular or intravenous administration, or both will be used. *The preparation for intramuscular injection* is given to multiple

sites, as soon as possible. The volume may be so large that anti-D immunoglobulin cannot be given without major discomfort to the patient. *The intravenous preparation* is given as an initial dose of 5 μg (25 i.u.) per ml of red cells and not exceeding 2500 μg (12 500 i.u.). The immunoglobulin is diluted in saline (500 ml) and administered slowly over one hour. Prior to infusion hydrocortisone 100 mg i.v. should be given. The infusion is repeated 12 hourly until the total calculated dose is given.

3. Monitoring the effect of anti-D immunoglobulin. Shivering, fever and haemoglobinuria may develop due to rapid clearance of Rh(D)-positive red cells. Good fluid intake and careful monitoring of fluid balance are essential. Antipyretics and antihistamines should be given.

Forty-eight hours after the administration of anti-D immunoglobulin, the Kleihauer test in TPH and serological tests following transfusion, should be repeated. If Rh(D)-positive cells are still in the circulation further doses of anti-D should be given, unti Rh(D)-positive cells cannot be demonstrated in the patient's blood. The patient should be recalled after six months to establish whether the antibody response has been prevented.

Some women may receive such a large volume of Rh(D)-positive red cells that an exchange transfusion must be carried out before anti-D immunoglobulin is administered.

The Kleihauer test and the calculation of the dose of anti-D immunoglobulin required to suppress immunisation

Films prepared from a sample of the mother's blood obtained immediately after birth are treated with an acid buffer. At low pH adult haemoglobin is soluble and is eluted from the red cells while fetal haemoglobin (Hb F) is insoluble and remains within the fetal red cells. On staining adult red cells appear as pale cell ghosts, whereas fetal red cells stain darkly. In over 90% of women the number of fetal red cells detected in the peripheral blood film immediately after delivery is less than 1 per 20 000 adult red cells (1 fetal red cell seen in 5 low-power fields). The standard dose of 100 μg (500 i.u.) of anti-D immunoglobulin is sufficient to remove from the circulation 4 ml of fetal red cells, the volume which on the peripheral blood film will give the ratio of 1 fetal red cell to 600 adult red cells. The size of feto-maternal bleed is calculated from the formula:

$$F = C \times f/a$$

where F is feto-maternal bleed in ml, C is a constant equal to 2400 and f and a are the numbers of fetal and adult red cells, respectively, in each low-power field. When using the formula an assumption that the mother's red cell mass is 1800 ml is made.

Example: In the peripheral blood film of a mother suspected of having TPH there are on average 10 fetal red cells and 2000 adult red cells in each low-power field. Feto-maternal bleed is:

$$F = 2400 \times 10/2000 = 12 \text{ ml}$$

The total dose of anti-D immunoglobulin required to remove all the fetal cells from the circulation is 12×25 μg $= 300$ μg (1500 i.u.).

Note that some women have congenitally high concentration of fetal haemoglobin in the blood and this may give rise to confusion in the Kleihauer test. Differential agglutination with saline anti-D immunoglobulin can be used to distinguish between the maternal and the baby's red cells with Hb F, whenever this condition is suspected.

REFERENCES

American Association of Blood Banks, Washington 1981 Blood components therapy. A physician's handbook, 3rd edn

Bussel B J, Hilgartner M W 1984 The use and mechanism of action of intravenous immunoglobulin in the treatment of immune haematological disease. British Journal of Haematology 56: 1–8

Cash J 1981 Blood replacement therapy. In: Bloom A L, Thomas D P (eds) Haemostasis and thrombosis. Churchill Livingstone, Edinburgh, ch 27, p 472–490

Department of Health and Social Security 1984 Notes on transfusion

Ingram G I C, Brozović M, Slater N G P 1982 Bleeding disorders. Investigation and management, 2nd edn. Blackwell Scientific, Oxford

Jones P 1979 Haemophilia management. A physician's guide to the treatment of haemophilia, Peter Jones and Travenol International Services

McClelland D B L, Yap P L 1984 Clinical use of immunoglobulins. In: Bayer W L (ed) Blood transfusion and blood banking. Clinics in haematology. Saunders, London, vol 13, p 39–74

Sherman L A 1984 New plasma components. In: Bayer W L (ed) Blood transfusion and blood banking. Clinics in haematology. Saunders, London, vol 13, p 17–38

WHO/IUIS Report 1982: Appropriate use of human immunoglobulins in clinical practice Bulletin of World Health Organization 60: 43–47

8. PLASMA SUBSTITUTES

Plasma substitutes are colloid and crystalloid solutions which are used for maintaining the circulatory volume following acute haemorrhage, shock, burns or septicaemia. Plasma substitutes have no oxygen carrying capacity and lack haemostatic properties. Crystalloid solutions have no plasma oncotic activity and colloid solutions possess it only temporarily as their half-life in the circulation is rather short. The use of plasma substitutes in an emergency 'buys time' necessary for provision of compatible blood and appropriate blood products. The main advantages and disadvantages of plasma substitutes are listed in Table 8.1.

Table 8.1 Advantages and disadvantages of colloid and crystalloid solutions

Solution	Advantages	Disadvantages
Crystalloids	readily available ease of storage ease of administration non-immunogenic non-toxic do not inhibit synthesis of albumin do not transmit diseases cheap	lack of oncotic pressure in plasma

Colloids	readily available
	ease of storage
	ease of administration
	do not transmit diseases
	provide oncotic pressure
	cheap
		short half-life in the circulation
		mildly immunogenic
		may interfere with haemostasis
		may interfere with blood grouping and
		  cross-matching
		may delay
		  replenishment of albumin

COLLOID SOLUTIONS

Dextrans

Definition
Polysaccharide fragments, slowly metabolised in the body, used to expand plasma volume.

Properties
Dextrans are mixtures of molecules with different molecular weights but in the preparations available the average molecular weight is standardised

Table 8.2 Main properties of dextrans

Name	Average molecular weight (Daltons)	Concentration in solution for infusion (g/dl)	Half-life in the circulation after infusion (hours)
Dextran 40	40 000	10	2–6
Dextran 70	70 000	6	6
Dextran 110	110 000	6	8
Dextran 150	150 000	6	8–10

(Table 8.2). Dextrans are available as solutions in 0.9% sodium chloride or 5% glucose in 500 ml bottles. Dextrans exert a colloidal osmotic pressure and draw extracellular fluid into the plasma. They also reduce plasma viscosity by reducing the fibrinogen concentration and the red cell count. Dextrans have an antithrombotic action through interfering with the platelet — factor VIII:vW — endothelial cell interaction. Dextrans are excreted via the kidney, smallest molecules first, thus the half-life in the circulation depends on the molecular size.

Storage and shelf-life
Dextrans are stored at room temperature and have a shelf-life of three to five years.

Indications for use and dosage
1. Conditions associated with peripheral local slowing of the blood flow. The initial dose is 500 to 1000 ml of Dextran 40, and further doses are administered on the individual merit of each case.
2. Blood volume expansion in burns. The dose is 500 to 1000 ml administered rapidly followed by further doses of up to a total of 3000 ml during the first few days. The oxygenation of tissues and electrolyte balance should not be forgotten.
3. Prophylaxis of post-operative thrombosis. The dose is 500 ml over four to six hours daily, or on alternate days, until the patient becomes mobile.
4. Dextran is used as a plasma substitute in plasma exchange and in extracorporeal circulation, mainly to reduce the requirement for fresh frozen plasma (FFP), plasma protein fraction (PPF) and blood.
5. Dextran can be used for harvesting granulocytes by apheresis (p. 157).

Note that dextrans should not be used as the only solution to expand and maintain the blood volume when shock is due to haemorrhage or severe sodium depletion.

Caution
Maintain hydration; improve oxygenation by giving blood or packed cells, and electrolyte balance by giving crystalloid solutions. Do not exceed the rate of administration of 500 ml/hour as allergic reactions and release of

histamine may occur. Do not administer more than 1500 ml in 24 hours and 3000 ml in the first few days.

Note that dextrans cause rouleaux formation, and blood samples for grouping and cross-matching must be collected before infusion is begun.

Contraindications
1. Congestive cardiac failure.
2. Renal failure with urea over 10 mmol/l and urinary output less than 1500 ml/24 hours.
3. Disseminated intravascular coagulation, bleeding diathesis and thrombocytopenia.

Side effects
1. Hypotension due to release of vasoactive substances.
2. Circulatory overload.
3. Rarely, anaphylactoid reactions, bronchospasm, rigors, urticaria.
4. Renal failure due to plugging of capillaries by the polysaccharide fragments.
5. Capillary oozing and bleeding tendency. In a patient with normal haemostasis this happens only when the volume of dextran infused exceeds 20 ml/kg body weight.

Hydroxyethyl starch

Definition
Hydroxyethyl starch (HES) is a colloid derived from a waxy starch, which after infusion, is slowly catabolised in the body.

Properties
HES contains modified amylopectin of molecular weight 450 000. It is a 6% solution in 0.9% sodium chloride. HES is slowly degraded in the body by amylase, partly excreted in the urine and partly taken up by the reticulo-endothelial system (RES). Its initial half-life in the circulation is 24 hours, but almost 20% of the infused HES remains in the body after one week.

Storage
HES is stored at room temperature.

Indications for use
1. Expansion of blood volume.
2. HES is used as an additive to increase granulocyte yields in leucapheresis by cell separators.

Caution
Concern has been expressed about the long term effects of HES remaining in the circulation and later in the RES. While this would be of limited importance to the patient who received only one infusion of HES, the significance of the cumulative effect of HES may be considerable when repetitive infusions are administered, as for example in leucapheresis donors.

Contraindication
Administration to patients with cardiac failure, renal failure or those who are severely dehydrated.
   Side effects are rare: circulatory overload, renal failure and mild bleeding tendency. Anaphylactic reactions are extremely rare.

Gelatin

Definition
A preparation of gelatin or partly degraded gelatin used to expand plasma volume.

Properties
Succinyl gelatin and partially degraded gelatin have molecular weight of 30 000. They are available as 3.5 to 4.0% solutions in 500 ml bottles (Gelofusine; Haemaccel). Gelatin has a half-life in the circulation of two to three hours, is completely metabolised in the body and the metabolites are excreted in the urine. Gelatin has no antigenic properties and does not influence haemostasis.

Storage and shelf-life
Gelatin preparations are stable at room temperature for up to eight years.

Indications for use and dosage
   1. Blood volume expansion, while awaiting compatible blood. The dose is 500 to 1000 ml.
   2. As a plasma substitute in plasma exchange and extracorporeal circulation. The total dose is up to 2000 ml, usually in combination with fresh frozen plasma (FFP) and plasma protein fraction (PPF).

Contraindication
Severe congestive cardiac failure.

Side effects
Inappropriately rapid administration of gelatin may cause the release of vasoactive substances, particularly dangerous in patients with allergic conditions such as asthma.

CRYSTALLOID SOLUTIONS

Definition
Crystalloid solutions are intravenous infusion fluids which usually contain a mixture of electrolytes.

Properties
The composition of crystalloid solutions, such as saline, Ringer's or Hartmann's solution are presented in Table 8.3. Crystalloid solutions have the capacity to expand the plasma volume, but only temporarily,

Table 8.3 Concentration of electrolytes in some intravenous fluids

Intravenous fluid	Concentration (mmol/l)				
	Na^+	K^+	HCO_3^-	Cl^-	Ca^{+2}
Normal plasma*	142+	4.5	26	103	2.5
Citrated plasma	150	12.0	—	55	—
Gelatin	145	5.1	—	145	6.2
Saline (normal)	150	—	—	150	—
Ringer's solution	147	4.0	—	156	2.2
Hartmann's solution	131	5.0	29	11	1.0

* Presented for comparison

since the intravascular and extravascular concentrations of electrolytes tend to equilibrate quickly. As the crystalloid solutions lack oncotic activity, judicial administration of fluids is required to avoid flooding of the extracellular space, and in particular, pulmonary oedema.

Storage and shelf-life

Crystalloid solutions are stored at room temperature and have a long shelf-life.

Indications for use and dose

1. Immediate treatment of haemorrhagic shock and burns until plasma protein fraction (PPF), albumin, fresh frozen plasma or blood are available. In haemorrhagic shock a volume of crystalloids two to three times greater than the estimated blood loss is generally used. Metabolic acidosis commonly accompanies shock and crystalloid solutions with some buffering capacity should be given.
2. Replacement solution in plasma exchange (p. 158).

Note that blood and appropriate blood component therapy should be given as soon as possible after infusion of large volumes of crystalloid solutions.

REFERENCES

British National Formulary 1984 British Medical Association and Pharmaceutical Society of Great Britain, Number 7
Collins J A, Murawiek K, Shafer A W (eds) 1982 Massive transfusion in surgery and trauma. Alan Liss, New York
Petz L D, Swisher S N 1981 Clinical practice of blood transfusion. Churchill Livingstone, New York
Smit Sibinga C T, Das P C, van Loghem J J 1982 Blood transfusion and problems of bleeding. Martinus Nijhof, The Hague

9. HAEMOLYTIC TRANSFUSION REACTIONS

HAEMOLYTIC TRANSFUSION REACTION

Definition
Destruction of red cells in the recipient's circulation arising as a direct result of transfusion of blood or blood components.

Pathogenesis
In most instances haemolysis is caused by an immune mechanism and the donor's cells are destroyed by the recipient's alloantibody, but occasionally the recipient's cells may be destroyed by an antibody present in the donor's plasma. Rarely, there may be an interaction between the red cells of one unit of blood and antibodies of another unit, transfused serially. Exceptionally, haemolysis occurs as a result of non-immune injury to red cells.

IMMUNE HAEMOLYTIC TRANSFUSION REACTION

Definition
The destruction of red cells in the recipient of a transfusion, caused by immune alloantibodies.

Pathogenesis
The type of haemolysis and the severity of a haemolytic transfusion reaction depend on the properties of the antibody involved.

1. A *direct cytotoxic effect* is exhibited by some antibodies which fix complement, whether IgG or IgM. Such antibodies bring about intravascular lysis of red cells. The stroma-antibody complexes cause a generalised Schwartzman reaction associated with disseminated intravascular coagulation, hypotension, shock and renal failure.

2. *Coating of red cells* by the corresponding antibody results in the rapid sequestration of the coated cells by the mononuclear phagocyte system (MPS) and phagocytosis by macrophages. This type of haemolysis (extravascular haemolysis) is usually found with IgG antibodies which do not bind complement. Destruction of red cells causes rigors,

muscle and joint pain, hyperbilirubinaemia,
haemoglobinaemia, haemoglobinuria and increasing anaemia.
The severity of the haemolytic reaction depends on the following
properties of alloantibodies.

Thermal amplitude: antibodies which do not react at 37°C are usually
harmless. *Antibody structure and complement fixation*: IgM antibodies are
more efficient in fixing complement and activating the complement
cascade than IgG antibodies, and are therefore more likely to have a
cytolytic effect. IgG antibodies usually coat red cells and provide the Fc
marker required for the onset of phagocytosis. IgG_1 and IgG_3 subclasses
of antibodies are rich in Fc marker, and are usually responsible for in
vivo haemolysis. *Haptenic structure*: most alloantibodies are directed
against glycoprotein or glycolipid structures; they generally react best at
25°C or lower temperatures and many fix complement. Antibodies in the
Rh system (p. 14) directed against a core protein antigen, usually react
at 37°C, rarely bind complement and frequently cause in vivo haemolysis.
The severity of the reaction also depends on the '*dose*' (amount) of the
incompatible blood transfusion, on the *concentration* and *avidity* of the
alloantibody and on the state of recipient's *MPS*. The main characteristics
of common alloantibodies are shown in Table 9.1.

Clinical presentation

Haemolytic transfusion reactions can be classified according to their
severity as severe, moderate and mild, and by their timing as immediate
or delayed.

Immediate haemolytic transfusion reaction

Severe haemolytic transfusion reaction

Anxiety, chest pain, back pain, headache, dyspnoea, rigors, vomiting,
diarrhoea, restlessness, tachycardia, hypotension, shock, unexplained
bleeding and renal shut down, occur in quick succession. In the
anaesthetised patient persistent hypotension and unexplained oozing from
the wound or needle puncture sites can be the only signs. The serum is
characteristically reddish brown due to free haemoglobin in serum, and
urine is dark due to haemoglobinuria.

Diagnosis is made by finding that the wrong unit of blood is being
transfused, on the basis of visual inspection of serum and urine, and on
the results of laboratory investigations shown in Table 9.2. Septicaemic
shock should be considered in differential diagnosis. For detailed
procedure of investigating suspected haemolytic transfusion reaction see
p. 92.

Management of severe haemolytic transfusion reaction

1. Stop transfusion immediately, keep i.v. line open with saline.
   Administer hydrocortisone 100 mg and an antihistamine (i.e.
   chlorpheniramine, Piriton, 10 mg) i.v.
2. Check labels on all units of blood and the name on all

Table 9.1 Some characteristics of common alloantibodies

In vitro behaviour	Thermal amplitude	Specificity	Ig class	In vivo behaviour
Agglutinating, sometimes haemolytic	below 25°C	Anti-P_1, -A_1, -M, -N, -Le^a	IgM	harmless
Coating	below 25°C	Anti-Xg^a, -Ch^a, -Rg^a, -Cs^a, -Sd^a, -Le^a	IgG	harmless
Coating	at 37°C	Anti-D, -c, -Fy^a, -K	IgG	extravascular haemolysis
Coating and complement fixing	at 37°C	Anti-Jk^a, -Fy^a	IgG	both intra- and extravascular lysis
Haemolytic, complement fixing	37°C and below	Anti-A, -B	IgM	severe intravascular haemolysis

Note that some alloantibodies appear in more than one category. Different individuals produce antibodies with different characteristics although of the same specificities

Table 9.2 Laboratory investigation and differential diagnosis of haemolytic transfusion reaction (HTR)

Type of reaction	Evidence for intravascular haemolysis				Evidence for extravascular haemolysis				Effect on haemostasis	
	Hb in serum	Hb in urine	Urobilinogen in urine	Hb conc.	Reticulocytes	DAT*	Spherocytes	Serum bilirubin	Platelet count	Coagulation screen
HTR, severe										
— early	+++	++	normal	→	normal	++	absent	normal	⇊→	abnormal
— late	++	+	⇈	⇊	↑	+++	±	↑		normal
HTR, moderate	±	+	⇈	⇊	↑	+++	++	⇈	normal	normal
HTR, delayed	absent	absent	↑	→	↑	+++	++	↑	normal	abnormal
Non-immune haemolysis	++	+	normal	→	normal	−	absent	normal	⇊	abnormal
Septicaemic or anaphylactic shock	absent	absent	normal	normal or ↓	normal	−	absent	normal	may be ↓	may be abnormal

* DAT, direct antiglobulin test
± present or absent; + mild; ++ moderate; +++ marked; ↑ increased; ⇈ markedly increased; ↓ decreased; ⇊ markedly decreased.

documentation to exclude error. Send all used blood packs or bottles, administration set, blood samples and urine sample to the blood bank (p. 93).
3. Start fluid balance chart. Give fluids intravenously (usually 1 litre saline per hour). If urinary output is below 100 ml per hour, give frusemide, 40 to 120 mg i.v. to maintain urinary flow. Whenever possible monitor CVP.
4. When there is any evidence of untoward bleeding or if laboratory tests indicate disseminated intravascular coagulation administer heparin 5000 i.u. intravenously. Larger or repeated doses of heparin are needed when over 200 ml of incompatible blood is transfused.
5. Maintain blood volume and urinary flow by giving PPF; when bleeding is present give FFP. Platelet concentrates are only needed when the count falls below $30 \times 10^9/l$. Dextrans are contraindicated.
6. If the urinary volume remains or becomes less than 100 ml per hour, repeat frusemide 40 to 120 mg i.v.
7. When the patient is profoundly anaemic and compatible blood or packed cells are available, continue with appropriate blood transfusion. Transfuse slowly, not more than one unit of blood every 12 hours.

Complications
1. Pulmonary oedema is usually due to fluid overload. Whenever possible monitor CVP. Reduce volume of fluids given (see also p. 102).
2. Progressive oliguria and renal failure. Refer the patient to specialist centre for dialysis.

Moderate haemolytic transfusion reaction
Anxiety, palpitations, mild dyspnoea, flushing, rigors, fever occur. If transfusion is continued while these symptoms and signs are present, it may develop into a severe reaction. Jaundice becomes apparent within two to 12 hours. Occasionally free haemoglobin is detected in urine.

Diagnosis is established on the basis of laboratory tests. Reaction to white cells, platelets or plasma proteins should be considered in differential diagnosis (p. 96).

Management
1. Stop transfusion, keep i.v. line open. Administer hydrocortisone 100 mg and an antihistamine i.v.
2. Check labels on all used blood units and all documentation, send all used units and fresh blood and urine samples to the laboratory.
3. Start fluid balance chart.
4. If the patient's condition remains unchanged repeat the dose of antihistamine.
5. Observe closely during the next three to four hours. If there is no evidence of hypotension and urinary output is

satisfactory, no further action is needed. If the condition does not improve, the management is as for severe haemolytic transfusion reaction.

Mild haemolytic transfusion reaction
This presents with a mild degree of fever and often passes unnoticed. It should be distinguished from non-haemolytic febrile transfusion reaction (NHFTR) usually associated with fever, pruritus, urticaria or slight abdominal pain. NHFTR is commonly due to alloantibodies to white cells, platelets or plasma proteins and is described on p. 96.

Delayed haemolytic transfusion reaction

Haemolysis of the transfused red cells in the recipient's circulation which occurs three to 21 days after transfusion is due to an anamnestic antibody response. Jaundice, progressive anaemia, fever, arthralgia and myalgia as well as a serum-sickness-like illness are commonly encountered. Delayed transfusion reactions may remain undetected, particularly in patients during the post-operative period. An anamnestic antibody response is most often directed against antigens in the Rh system. Most patients have been previously exposed to these antigens (pregnancy, previous transfusions) and produce a brisk anamnestic response with IgG antibodies.

Diagnosis
Once suspected, the diagnosis is easily established by
1. a positive direct antiglobulin test (DAT), given by some cells in the patient's circulation (mixed field appearance) (see p. 189).
2. on the basis of a positive antibody screen. The identification of the antibody is usually easy. When the DAT and antibody screen are negative other causes of jaundice with fever and arthralgia, such as viral hepatitis, obstructive jaundice and the resorption of large haematomata must be considered.

Management
Symptomatic treatment with oral antipyretics (aspirin 300 to 600 mg t.d.s.) and/or antihistamines (chlorpheniramine, Piriton, 10 mg b.d. or t.d.s.) are used. Avoid transfusion unless anaemia is profound, as an anamnestic antibody response to a different antigen may occur.

Prevention of haemolytic transfusion reactions

Severe haemolytic transfusion reactions carry a high mortality, but fortunately they occur rarely. The majority of such transfusion catastrophes are due to preventable clerical or technical errors, for example: collecting the blood sample for cross-matching from the wrong patient, giving blood to the wrong patient, recording the wrong blood group or the wrong patient's name. These errors of identification, transcription and omission can only be prevented by careful attention to detail, particularly when identifying the patient. Each hospital blood bank should have 'specification of procedures' (SOP) describing the collection of blood for blood grouping and compatibility testing, serological testing and record keeping, issue of blood and blood components and their administration on the wards. SOPs should contain all the recommendations set out in 'Notes on transfusion' (DHSS, 1984).

Transfusion in patients known to have alloantibodies

When transfusing a patient with alloantibodies, sufficient time must be allowed for the blood bank to identify the antibody(s) and to find compatible blood. The patient who has once produced an alloantibody is likely to do so again, and *to a different antigen.*

It is sometimes impossible to find compatible blood quickly for a patient with multiple alloantibodies. If the blood is required for an elective procedure and there is time in hand, several options are available:

1. *autotransfusion* by leap-frogging or with frozen and thawed red cells (p. 43);
2. *phenotyping members of the family* to find one who is lacking the same antigen as the patient;
3. *searching for compatible donors* on the national and international panels of rare blood group donors. In the U.K. this should be done in the first instance through the Regional Transfusion Centre. If further help is necessary it can be obtained from the Blood Group Reference Laboratory in Oxford, where the national and international files of donors with rare blood groups are held, and the European Bank of Frozen Blood of Rare Groups in Amsterdam; and when all the previous measures have failed, by
4. *measuring in vivo survival of ^{51}Cr labelled incompatible cells.* It is occasionally possible to show that incompatible cells survive in the patient for two to three weeks, and that such incompatible blood can be transfused safely.

Emergency transfusion in patients with alloantibodies for whom no compatible blood is available at the time

The doctor in charge of the patient, after consultation with the haematologist, must decide at what stage the danger of anaemia or exsanguination becomes greater than the danger of a possible transfusion reaction. If it is decided to give incompatible blood, the blood can only be issued at the doctor's explicit request and after signing a special form. The following procedure should be followed:

1. Administer hydrocortisone 100 mg and chlorpheniramine (Piriton) 10 mg i.v. prior to transfusion of each unit. Transfuse slowly (one unit a day) and through an in-line blood warmer. Use washed, frozen and thawed or packed red cells. If none are available use stored blood to minimize the complement content of plasma.

2. Observe the patient quarter-hourly. Keep a fluid balance chart. Check urine for free haemoglobin.
3. Slow down or stop transfusion if any untoward effects occur.
4. Check patient's haemoglobin concentration at the end of transfusion to see whether the expected rise has been achieved.
5. Check bilirubin and haemoglobin in serum and urine, as well as blood count.

Transfusion of patients with anti-Le^a and anti-Le^b antibodies

Most anti-Le antibodies are not active at 37°C and are not harmful in vivo. Patients with *warm* anti-Le^a antibodies should be given Le(a–) blood. If such blood is not available, or if the patient has both anti-Le^a and –Le^b (Le(a–b–) blood may be difficult to find*), he or she can be given Le-incompatible cells provided the administration of blood is preceded by the transfusion of one or two units of AB secretor plasma (see pp. 9, 64). The Le^a and Le^b substance in the plasma neutralises the antibody(ies) and the red cells can be given safely. If secretor plasma is not available, the patient should be transfused with whole blood, rather than packed cells, for the Le substance in the donor's plasma will partly neutralise the recipient's antibody. The procedure described on p. 90 should be followed during the transfusion.

Other reasons for immune haemolysis

Transfusion of incompatible plasma

Patients of blood group A, B or AB, receiving O blood with a high titre IgG anti-A or anti-B reacting at 37°C, donated by the 'dangerous universal donor' (p. 9) may experience a moderate transfusion reaction, with jaundice and progressive anaemia. Immune anti-A and anti-B are sometimes responsible for haemolysis following administration of large amounts of blood products (p. 68).

Donor plasma containing anti-D, anti-K or other alloantibodies, may inadvertently be transfused. Mild to moderate haemolysis with mild jaundice, spherocytosis, a positive DAT and a fall in haemoglobin concentration are the usual manifestations.

Incompatibility between two donor units

In rare instances the incompatibility is due to an antibody present in one unit of blood affecting the red cells from the other unit. The recipient experiences mild haemolysis.

Diagnosis

Routine investigation for a haemolytic transfusion reaction usually discloses the cause of haemolysis (p. 92).

The management of haemolytic transfusion reaction is described on p. 88.

---

* In ethnic groups with a high incidence of Le(a–b–) phenotype this should not present a problem.

NON-IMMUNE HAEMOLYTIC TRANSFUSION REACTION

Transfusion of haemolysed blood
Blood can be haemolysed if it is infected, heated over 50°C, passed under pressure through a narrow orifice or frozen (usually if the refrigerator temperature falls below –3°C). Transfusion of one or more units of lysed blood is extremely dangerous because it can cause severe haemolytic reaction with DIC, hypotensive shock and renal failure.

Diagnosis
Visual inspection of the unit of blood containing sedimented red cells or after centrifugation will show that the plasma is dark. For details of diagnostic procedure see the end of this chapter; for findings in the recipient see Table 9.2.

Management is the same as for severe transfusion reaction. If haemolysis is due to bacterial contamination additional measures described on p. 122 are required.

Haemolysis due to osmotic lysis
Blood mixed with 5% dextrose undergoes osmotic lysis and may give rise to a severe transfusion reaction. Osmotic lysis can also be caused by the injection of water into the circulation. It usually occurs after prostatectomy when the bladder is irrigated with water instead of saline. Severe intravascular haemolysis occurs associated with hyponatraemia and hypokalaemia. It carries a high mortality.

The diagnosis is established by careful investigation of transfusion procedures, in the absence of abnormal serological findings. For details see the end of this chapter.

Management is the same as for a severe transfusion reaction (p. 86). Electrolyte balance should be restored as soon as possible.

Transfusion of 'old' blood
Transfusion of large amounts of blood near the expiry date may provoke hyperbilirubinaemia and fever. The recipient's haemoglobin fails to reach the expected level. The serum bilirubin may rise rapidly to reach a maximum on the first day, or gradually over the next four to five days.

Diagnosis is by exclusion of other reasons for haemolysis (and finding that the units transfused were near the expiry date).

Management
Symptomatic treatment only is required. Transfuse with fresh blood if anaemia is profound.

INVESTIGATION OF A SUSPECTED HAEMOLYTIC TRANSFUSION REACTION

Action at the bedside
   1. Inspect urine for presence of haemoglobin. If haemoglobin is present the colour is altered: depending on the concentration

of haemoglobin it varies from pink through brownish to almost black.

2. Send to the laboratory: the blood unit implicated and all empty bags (if any unit was previously given); the administration set used; 20 ml clotted blood for serological tests, blood in a sequestrene tube for blood count including platelet count and in a citrate tube for coagulation tests; urine sample.
3. Take blood cultures.
4. Always check the patient's name against the name on the blood units and in the transfusion record, as well as the name on all tubes of blood sent for testing.
5. Check transfusion procedures to exclude mechanical, osmotic or other non-immune reasons for haemolysis.
6. Interpret the results of laboratory tests according to Table 9.2.

Action in the blood bank
1. Re-check, jointly with the ward, for the possibility of an error.
2. Repeat the blood group determination on the recipient's pre- and post-transfusion blood and all units of blood used.
3. Re-cross-match all units of blood used against pre- and post-transfusion blood samples.
4. Carry out antibody screen on both pre- and post-transfusion serum.
5. If an antibody is detected, identify it and search for compatible units.
6. If no immune mechanism is detected, transfusion procedures must be re-checked. Consult flow chart on Table 9.3.

Table 9.3 Flow chart for investigation of a suspected haemolytic transfusion reaction

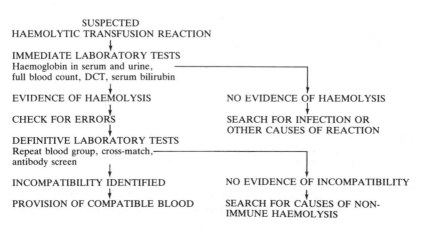

REFERENCES

Department of Health and Social Security 1984 Notes on transfusion

Greenwalt T J 1981 Pathogenesis and management of hemolytic transfusion reactions. In: Conrad M E (ed) Transfusion problems in hematology. Seminars in Hematology 18: 84–94

Mollison P L 1983 Blood transfusion in clinical medicine, 7th edn. Blackwell Scientific, Oxford

Petz L D, Swisher S N (eds) 1981 Clinical practice of blood transfusion. Churchill Livingstone, Edinburgh

10. NON-HAEMOLYTIC IMMUNE TRANSFUSION REACTIONS

Non-haemolytic immune transfusion reactions are brought about by the action of alloantibodies, present in the circulation of the sensitised recipient, and corresponding antigenic determinants on leucocytes, platelets or plasma immunoglobulins transfused. A large proportion of these reactions are due to HLA antibodies, since the sensitising episodes are comparatively frequent, e.g. pregnancy and blood transfusion, and viable lymphocytes are present almost invariably in red cell, platelet and granulocyte preparations. The remaining small proportion of the reactions are due to antibodies to specific granulocyte and platelet antigens and antigenic determinants on immunoglobulins.

REACTIONS TO LEUCOCYTES

Transfusion reactions to leucocytes are the result of an antigen-antibody reaction where the antigen involved is either one of the HLA antigens or granulocyte-specific. The reaction activates complement which in turn causes lysis of granulocytes with liberation of pyrogens as well as the release of various vasoactive substances; fever and/or urticarial and anaphylactic reactions may ensue.

Alloimmunisation to leucocyte antigens
The frequency with which antibodies to granulocytes develop is high and it is proportional to the number of exposures. Multiparous women are often sensitised to leucocyte antigens, presumably through transplacental leakage of fetal blood: four to 25% of women after two pregnancies, and over 50% after three pregnancies are sensitised. Almost 90% of recipients of massive transfusion, multiple transfusions or granulocyte transfusions develop either anti-HLA or antibodies to granulocytes. The antibody(ies) is usually apparent one week after transfusion. It should not be assumed that all sensitised patients will experience transfusion reactions when they receive blood and blood products. However, in the majority of those who do have an overt transfusion reaction, antibodies to HLA antigens and/or to granulocyte specific antigens can be demonstrated.

Non-haemolytic febrile transfusion reaction (NHFTR)

Definition and pathological physiology

A febrile episode occurs half an hour to two hours after the onset of transfusion. The reaction is due to pyrogens, released from the granulocytes damaged by complement in an antigen-antibody reaction. Leucocytes can also be damaged mechanically, for example as a consequence of leucapheresis, especially filtration leucapheresis.

Clinical picture

The most severe NHFTR presents with a rise of temperature to over 39°C associated with flushing, palpitations and tachycardia, followed by headache and rigors. If the transfusion is continued, or if the reaction is very severe, cough, breathlessness and respiratory distress may ensue. Some patients develop an urticarial rash and/or angioneurotic oedema at the same time.

In a less severe reaction, chills and rise in temperature may be the only symptom and sign. In the mildest form of NHFTR the patient remains asymptomatic and there is only a rise in temperature not exceeding 38°C. In general, the height and the duration of fever are proportional to the number of leucocytes transfused ('antigenic load'), and the fever usually lasts between two and 12 hours.

Diagnosis and differential diagnosis

A diagnosis of NHFTR, made clinically, can be confirmed only by laboratory tests showing absence of haemolysis, and thus excluding haemolytic transfusion reaction (p. 92). Coincidental infection should be also considered in the differential diagnosis. Ideally, the cause of NHFTR should be established. In practice, only patients receiving multiple transfusions are investigated for the presence of antibodies to granulocytes and to HLA antigens. *Note* that immune reactions to platelets and/or plasma proteins may also provoke the release of pyrogenic substances and febrile reaction.

Management

1. Slow down, or in a severe reaction, stop the transfusion of blood.
2. Keep the i.v. line open by saline drip, keep the patient warm, and collect blood samples to exclude a haemolytic transfusion reaction. Return the blood units to the blood bank.
3. Administer aspirin or paracetamol to combat the fever. In patients with severe symptoms 100 mg of hydrocortisone i.v. can also be given. Antihistamines do not affect the fever, but may be used to suppress a concomitant urticaria or anaphylactoid reaction.
4. Observe the patient closely at 15 or 30 min intervals.
5. If the patient requires further transfusion(s), send blood samples for antibody screen and compatibility testing (p. 185, 187), and later, for detection of leucoagglutinins and HLA antibodies (p. 47).

Prevention
NHFTR may be prevented by transfusing leucocyte depleted blood or suppressed by drugs.

1. *Leucocyte depleted blood* (p. 25). Multitransfused patients with a history of NHFTR should receive blood filtered using a microaggregate filter, at the bedside. Should this simple measure be ineffective in abolishing NHFTR, blood depleted of leucocytes by buffy coat removal, red cell washing, sedimentation or filtration with leucocyte depleting filters, should be administered. Frozen and thawed red cells are usually reserved for patients in whom other methods of leucocyte depletion have failed to abolish NHFTR. Such patients should *always* be tested for antibodies to leucocytes as well as for anti-IgA (p. 98).

2. *Suppression* is used when leucocyte depleted blood is not available, and for patients receiving platelet and granulocyte concentrates, who have a history of febrile reactions in the past. Usually antihistamines (chlorpheniramine, Piriton, 10 mg) and hydrocortisone (100 mg i.v.) are given 15 or 30 min before transfusion. Aspirin, 300 mg, can also be given to recipients who do not have a bleeding tendency.

General measures
Keep the patient warm and ordinarily do not exceed a transfusion rate of 500 ml per hour, because rapid transfusion increases the chance of having a febrile reaction.

Pulmonary infiltration
This term refers to radiographic findings of multiple nodular infiltrates in the lungs associated, in severe cases, with respiratory insufficiency. The syndrome is common with granulocyte transfusions, but occurs rarely when other kinds of blood and blood products are administered. The pathological physiology, clinical picture, diagnosis and management are described in Chapter 6.

Prevention
Always transfuse leucocyte depleted blood to patients with a history of febrile reactions, or to those known to have antibodies to leucocytes.

Graft versus host disease (GVHD)
Engraftment of donor lymphocytes may occur in severely immunosuppressed or immunodeficient individuals, as well as in premature babies. In most instances the only manifestation is a temporary graft of donor cells, recognized by their markers (the ABO group, G-6-PD isoenzymes, etc.). GVHD, although rare, has been described in a number of well documented cases.

Prevention
To abolish the capacity of immunocompetent lymphocytes it is recommended that blood, granulocyte and platelet concentrates are irradiated with 1500 to 3000 rad (15 to 30 Gy) before administration to severely immunocompromised recipients.

REACTIONS TO PLATELETS

These reactions are also due to the interaction between antigens on the platelets and corresponding antibodies. The result of the antigen-antibody reaction is the destruction of transfused platelets and, less commonly, febrile or anaphylactoid reactions.

Alloimmunisation to platelet antigens
About 70% of patients who have received 10 to 20 units of random donor platelet concentrates develop antibodies to HLA or platelet specific antigens within one to two weeks after transfusion. Patients receiving massive or multiple transfusions as well as multiparous women, develop antibodies to platelets.

Platelet refractoriness
Platelet refractoriness is the term used to describe the failure of platelet transfusion to raise the platelet count in the recipient. It represents the most serious manifestation of alloimmunisation to platelet antigens (p. 57).

Febrile reactions
Febrile reactions after platelet transfusions are usually caused by pyrogens released from leucocytes. For management and prevention see p. 96.

Anaphylactoid reactions
Anaphylactoid reactions are common (p. 99).

Granulocytopenia
Severe granulocytopenia is sometimes encountered with HLA incompatible platelet transfusion. It may persist for up to 48 hours.

Post-transfusion purpura
Acute thrombocytopenia occurring one week after transfusion is called post-transfusion purpura (p. 146).

REACTIONS TO PLASMA PROTEINS

Transfusion reactions associated with plasma proteins are urticaria and anaphylactoid reactions, although febrile reactions and reactions due to passive transfer of antibodies also occur.

Alloimmunisation to plasma proteins
1. Antibodies to antigenic determinants on IgG molecules of different subclasses arise as a consequence of multiple transfusions (thalassaemia major), exchange transfusion (haemolytic disease of the newborn), or exposure to blood products (e.g. haemophiliacs), as well as during pregnancy. The immunised individual lacks one of the IgG subclasses.
2. Antibodies to IgA are usually encountered in IgA deficient

individuals. The incidence of IgA deficient individuals is about 1 in 3000.

3. Up to 20% of multiply transfused patients may have antibodies to antigenic determinants on IgM molecules.

Urticaria

Definition and pathological physiology
Urticaria is one of the commmonest transfusion reactions and consists of circumscribed areas of cutaneous oedema. It is caused by the degranulation of mast cells in the skin and subsequent release of histamine. The degranulation is brought about by complement activation following the formation of immune complexes. The antigens commonly implicated are those on IgG and IgA, but antigens to leucocytes or platelets may also give rise to urticaria.

Clinical picture
Itching, widespread or localised rash with or without well defined margins are the usual manifestations.

Diagnosis
Urticaria is easily recognisable clinically.

Management
Slow down the transfusion, or stop if urticaria is severe. Administer an antihistamine (e.g. chlorpheniramine, Piriton, 10 mg). The rash usually subsides within 30 min. If no other signs of anaphylactoid reaction are observed, it is probably safe to continue with transfusion at a slow rate.

Prevention
Urticaria is a common and mild reaction which is not usually investigated, and does not require preventive measures. If, however, a patient experiences severe urticaria with each transfusion of blood or blood components, it is advisable to search for antibodies to plasma proteins. When the patient requires blood, washed red cells or frozen and thawed red cells, free of plasma proteins, can be used. For IgA deficient recipients with anti-IgA, blood and blood components collected from IgA deficient donors should be used.

Urticaria is also successfully prevented if an antihistamine (chlorpheniramine, Piriton) is given either one to two hours before transfusion or more conveniently, intravenously via the drip line over 15 to 30 sec at the beginning of the transfusion.

Anaphylactoid reaction

Definition and pathological physiology
Anaphylactoid reaction is a term used to describe an immediate hypersensitivity reaction. In susceptible individuals an antigen (in the case of blood and blood products, usually a determinant on serum immunoglobulins, or less commonly on white cells or platelets) provokes the production of antibodies to IgE. On subsequent exposure the antigen-antibody complex is formed on the surface of mast cells and basophilic

granulocytes leading to degranulation and release of various mediators, including histamine. These vasoactive substances cause bronchospasm, vasodilation, increased vascular permeability and hypotension, as well as vomiting and diarrhoea.

Clinical picture

The clinical manifestations of anaphylaxis vary from mild erythema to a rapid onset syndrome of hypotension and shock carrying a high mortality. In a mild reaction, erythema, pruritus, urticaria and angio-oedema of lips, tongue and eyelids are common. In more severe reactions respiratory problems are prominent: they may be due to upper airway obstruction by the oedema of larynx or epiglottis, or to lower airway obstruction caused by bronchospasm. Vomiting, diarrhoea and abdominal pain are also common. The most severe clinical manifestations are hypotension and shock due to peripheral vasodilation and increased vascular permeability.

Diagnosis

Because of rapid onset and potential seriousness, the diagnosis should be made clinically and management initiated promptly. Septic shock and severe haemolytic transfusion reaction should be considered in the differential diagnosis of severe reaction (p. 86).

Managment

Severe reaction

Stop the procedure, keep the drip line open with saline, raise the feet, administer 0.5 mg of adrenalin intramuscularly or 0.2 μg/kg body weight per minute intravenously. Repeat administration of adrenalin every 15 min until an improvement is seen. Chlorpheniramine (Piriton) 10 mg i.v. is a useful adjunct. Upper airway obstruction must be differentiated from diffuse bronchospasm. Severe laryngeal or epiglottal oedema may require endotracheal intubation, whereas bronchospasm is treated by inhalation of a β_2 adrenoceptor stimulant e.g. salbutamol or by intravenous aminophylline 5 mg/kg by slow intravenous injection. Severe hypotensive reactions require volume replacement and intensive resuscitation and monitoring best provided in an intensive care unit.

Moderate and mild reactions

Treat as for urticaria. If there is any evidence of airway obstruction treat as severe.

Prevention

Any patient who has experienced a severe anaphylatoid reaction after administration of blood or blood components should only receive washed or frozen and thawed red cells. Every attempt should be made to identify the antibody(ies) responsible. The most severe reactions are usually found in IgA deficient subjects who have developed anti-IgA. Some authorities believe that steroids administered before transfusion protect the recipient from anaphylactoid reactions.

Hypersensitivity reactions due to passively transfused antibody

Blood collected from donors who display strong hypersensitivity to a variety of antigens (in foods, pollen, drugs, etc.) may cause an immediate hypersensitivity reaction if the recipient had been exposed to the antigen involved at the time of blood transfusion. Urticaria, bronchospasm and reactions to penicillin due to this mechanism have been described in recipients of blood.

REFERENCES

Barton J C 1981 Nonhemolytic, noninfectious transfusion reactions. In: Conrad M E (ed) Transfusion problems in hematology. Seminars in Hematology 18: 95–121

Mollison P L 1983 Blood transfusion in clinical medicine, 7th edn. Blackwell Scientific Publications, Oxford

Petz L D, Swisher S N (eds) 1981 Clinical practice of blood transfusion. Churchill Livingstone, Edinburgh

11. OTHER REACTIONS TO BLOOD AND BLOOD COMPONENTS

CIRCULATORY OVERLOAD

Definition and pathological physiology
Circulatory overload follows either a rapid transfusion of blood, or a transfusion to recipients with impaired cardiac function and low cardiac reserve. The expansion of the circulatory blood volume by transfused blood leads to raised central venous pressure and to left ventricular failure with pulmonary congestion and oedema.

Clinical presentation
Circulatory overload may be immediate (during transfusion) or delayed for up to 24 hours after transfusion. Restlessness, headache, non-productive cough and tightness across the chest are the usual symptoms. In severe cases dyspnoea, orthopnea, tachycardia, cyanosis and chest pain occur; death may occur as a result of post-transfusion circulatory overload. On examination the patient has raised JVP and bilateral basal rales; hypertension, enlarged heart and gallop rhythm are common findings. Radiographic findings include: large heart, prominent pulmonary arteries and septal lines; in severe cases diffuse clouding of both lung fields is seen.

Management
Stop all intravenous fluids, administer diuretics (40 mg frusemide i.v. if none has been given prior to transfusion, or add additional diuretics). Sit the patient upright. In severe cases venesect the patient and withdraw 200 to 500 ml of blood. Digitalisation, oxygen and morphine may be required.

Prevention
This complication arises most commonly in patients with severe chronic anaemia (i.e. iron deficiency or megaloblastic anaemia) in a stable high output state, who are given blood transfusion. Such patients should, whenever possible, be allowed to respond to specific therapy and should *not* be transfused unless there is major organ failure (myocardial infarction, CVA, severe infection or intractable cardiac failure). If transfusion must be given, always use packed red cells, one unit a day, given over eight hours and preceded by frusemide 40 mg, orally or intravenously. The patient should be kept warm, in an upright position, and observed closely.

In very ill patients it may be safer to transfuse blood while monitoring CVP. If that is not possible, removal of 200 to 300 ml of blood by venesection before transfusion may prevent severe pulmonary oedema.

Other patients at risk are the multitransfused individuals with thalassaemia or sickle cell disease, whose cardiac function may be compromised by iron overload, and the elderly with heart conditions. The use of packed red cells, slow rate of transfusion and diuretics will prevent circulatory overload in the majority of such patients.

METABOLIC EFFECTS OF BLOOD TRANSFUSION

Citrate toxicity

Pathological physiology
Blood collected into ACD or CPD contains 1.4 to 1.6 g of citrate in a unit of blood. When massive or exchange transfusions are given, the toxic levels of citrate in plasma (about 100 mg/dl) can easily be reached.

In adults citrate toxicity is observed when the rate of transfusion is 1 l or more per 10 min, or when the amount transfused exceeds 6 l, or when an exchange transfusion is carried out in under two hours.

In infants citrate toxicity can occur during exchange transfusion (p. 34). Excess citrate in plasma binds and chelates the ionised calcium and all the symptoms and signs of citrate toxicity are due to hypocalcaemia.

Clinical features
Involuntary muscle tremors are usually the first and only warning signs. Cardiac arrythmias and ventricular fibrillation may supervene quickly. The ECG shows ST segment prolongation and T wave delay.

Management
If muscle tremors are observed, or if the transfusion rate exceeds 500 ml per 10 min, or if more than 5 l have been transfused to an adult (or one blood volume replaced in a child), an injection of 2.25 mmol of calcium (10 ml of 10% calcium gluconate for injection) should be administered i.v. It is essential to monitor plasma Ca^{+2} levels and ECG in such patients since hypercalcaemia may develop with equally dangerous consequences.

Prevention
Infants, patients with liver disease or those undergoing liver surgery are at particular risk from citrate toxicity. The following measures can be undertaken to minimise the risk.
1. Use of heparinised blood (p. 24 and 35).
2. Use of packed red cells (much of the citrate used for anticoagulation is removed with plasma).
3. Avoidance of hypothermia and hyperkalaemia, which potentiate citrate toxicity.

4. Prophylactic administration of calcium as described above. Remember that over-zealous use of calcium can also cause fatal cardiac arrest.

Potassium toxicity

Pathological physiology
Potassium toxicity occurs in massive transfusion; it must be considered in conjunction with citrate toxicity. The potassium load of stored blood increases with the length of storage (p. 22 and table 2.4) and after two weeks of storage each unit contains between 4 and 7 mmol of potassium. Hyperkalaemia alters cardiac excitability and can cause cardiac standstill.

Clinical picture and diagnosis
Potassium toxicity is suspected on the basis of abnormal ECG findings and confirmed by finding a high plasma potassium concentration.

Management
Prompt correction of hypocalcaemia due to citrate is essential.

Prevention
For patients with impaired renal function or after massive injury, use the freshest blood available (always less than ten days old). Use packed red cells in preference to whole blood.

Acid load

Pathological physiology
Blood collected into ACD or CPD anticoagulant has a significant base deficit: the pH of freshly collected ACD blood is 7.0, and of CPD blood is 7.2. After two weeks of storage the pH falls to 6.5 and 6.8, respectively. Massive transfusion with stored blood may aggravate the acidosis of shock or renal failure already present in the recipient. Hours after transfusion the citrate is converted into bicarbonate and can produce metabolic alkalosis.

Management
Administration of alkali is only required in an already acidotic patient. Whenever possible determine the 'base deficit' before giving bicarbonate, as excess sodium may aggravate the late alkalosis.

Prevention
Avoid use of blood stored for over two weeks in recipients at risk from developing acidosis.

Transfusion iron overload

Pathological physiology
Each unit of blood contains about 250 mg of iron. Because the excretion of iron in man is minimal and unless there is continuous blood loss,

transfusion of 100 to 150 units of blood will cause accummulation of 20 to 30 g of iron in the stores (compared to normal amount of 2 to 4 g). Iron is deposited in almost all organs and causes cell damage by two different mechanisms: iron catalyses the peroxidation of membrane lipids leading to cell destruction, and haemosiderin deposited in lysosymes renders them unstable and causes release of enzymes with subsequent cell damage and death.

The clinical picture resembles that of idiopathic haemochromatosis. Target organs of transfusion haemosiderosis (iron overload) are the liver, the endocrine glands, the heart and the skin. Liver dysfunction progresses to cirrhosis and liver failure; hypogonadism and diabetes are common. The caridac manifestations are pericarditis, chronic cardiac failure and cardiac arrhythmias. The skin becomes heavily pigmented.

Management and prevention (See also p. 33). It is important to start chelation therapy as early as possible: in transfusion dependent children preferably before the age of five. Desferrioxamine (Desferal) is administered as an intermittent subcutaneous infusion, 1 to 4 g 12 hourly, four to six times a week, or as a slow i.v. infusion lasting three to five days every four to six weeks. The dose should be determined individually on the basis of iron excretion. Vitamin C, 150 to 250 mg, is sometimes also given to assist the mobilisation of tissue iron, but it must be used with caution because it may increase iron toxicity to the heart in patients with severe iron overload.

Vasoactive substances

Pathological physiology
Various vasoactive substances may be found in stored blood and sometimes in FFP and plasma products. The presence of adenine, angiotensin, a bradykinin-like peptide released by kallikrein activated on cold storage, a peptide with vasoconstricting properties released from senescent platelets and a permeability factor liberated on fragmentation of factor XII (Hageman factor), have all been described.

Clinical picture
Several 'vasoactive' syndromes are described:
1. Hypotension, nausea, sweating and chest pain may occur after infusion of FFP and certain batches of PPF.
2. Failure of plasma volume expansion can be occasionally seen after PPF and FFP due to increased vascular permeability and leakage of plasma into the extravascular space.
3. Transient hypertension in the absence of circulatory overload has been described.

Management is symptomatic; the transfusion of blood or blood component must be stopped.

A hypertension-convulsion syndrome (see also p. 33) has been encountered in multitransfused patients with thalassaemia and sickle cell disease. Severe hypertension (particularly diastolic), headache, convulsions and subarachnoid haemorrhage occur one to 12 days after transfusion. The mortality, once the syndrome has occurred, is high.

The possibility of hypertension-convulsion syndrome must be kept in mind in multitransfused patients complaining of headache or whose diastolic blood pressure is over 90 mm Hg at the end of transfusion. Antihypertensive therapy, rest, and venesection if there is any evidence of circulatory overload or hyperviscosity are the only measures of prevention available. Anticonvulsant therapy should be given promptly to patients with fits.

Haemostatic defects

Haemostatic defects associated with massive transfusion are described on p. 38.

TRANSFUSION OF COLD BLOOD

Pathological physiology
Blood taken from the refrigerator and rapidly transfused without warming may cause profound hypothermia with oesophageal temperatures as low as 27°C. The effects of hypothermia are:

1. *Cardiac arrhythmias*, usually ventricular which may lead to cardiac arrest.
2. *Aggravation of citrate toxicity*.
3. *Reduction in the oxygen carrying capacity* of stored blood. Cold blood shows further shift to the left of the O_2 dissociation curve already affected by the reduction in the red cell 2,3-DPG concentration (p. 21).
4. *Painful venous spasm* is a common local problem when cold blood is transfused.

Clinical picture
Cardiac arrhythmia is the most prominent feature, particularly if the transfusion rate exceeds 50 ml/min.

Management and prevention
If arrythmia occurs, stop transfusion, warm the patient and transfuse blood through a warmer. It is important to use a blood warmer in emergencies where large volumes have to be transfused quickly to keep pace with bleeding.

PARTICULATE AND SOLUBLE FOREIGN MATTER

Pathological physiology
Particles and fibres from nylon or cellulose filters, glass fragments and pieces of rubber (when rubber stoppered glass bottles were used) have

been found in the circulation following transfusion. In experimental animals particulate matter causes lung microembolisation and fibrosis, but no such effects have been observed in humans.

Stringent quality control has abolished the use of those plastic containers for blood and blood components which released toxic substances on storage. Nevertheless, small amounts of plasticisers, used in the production of PVC catheters and containers, may be slowly dissolved in plasma lipids and may enter the recipient's circulation to become permanently deposited in the abdominal fat. It is unclear whether plasticisers have any adverse effects on humans, but it has been postulated that they play a role in the necrotizing enterocolitis which may follow neonatal exchange transfusion through PVC catheters.

MICROAGGREGATES

Pathological physiology
Microaggregates are clumps of fibrin, platelets and leukocytes, over 20 μm in diameter, which form in stored blood (see also p. 22). Platelet fibrinogen appears to be the primary determinant of microaggregate formation, although plasma fibrinogen also contributes to their formation. The presence of these particles markedly increases the screen filtration pressure of stored blood (the pressure needed to force the blood through a 20 μm filter at a constant rate).

Microaggregates form quickly on storage to reach a maximum number within one to two weeks. Some microaggregates will disaggregate thereafter, but a significant proportion will remain. When microaggregates enter the recipient's circulation, they are caught in the lungs where they may disaggregate, release the lysosomes from disintegrating cells which they contain and contribute to the mechanism of the adult respiratory distress syndrome seen after massive injury.

Prevention
The evidence that microaggregates are an etiological factor in ARDS is equivocal. Nevertheless, it is prudent to use microaggregate filters when patients are receiving massive transfusion and are at risk of developing shock lung (p. 37).

LOSS OF CATHETERS INTO VEINS

Many instances of loss of catheters (tips or other parts) have been recorded. The catheter travels to the right heart and is eventually embolised in the lungs.

When a catheter is lost into a vein, the vein should immediately be compressed proximally to the insertion site to prevent the escape of the

catheter. Immediate help from surgeons or anaesthetists should be sought
to remove the catheter locally. Once in the thorax the catheter can only
be removed by an open procedure. The problem can be prevented by
using appropriate needles or catheters with intravenous guides.

AIR EMBOLISM

Pathological physiology
Venous air embolism is nowadays a rare complication because the blood
is collected and stored in air-free, collapsible plastic bags; earlier it was
seen occasionally with rapid transfusion from glass bottles. As little as
10 ml of air can cause death due to sudden obstruction of the pulmonary
vasculature.
   Arterial air embolism is not a complication of blood transfusion; it
occurs as a rare complication of cardiac surgery, arterial punctures or
some arterial wounds. The air is trapped in the cerebrovascular
circulation and its sudden obstruction causes convulsions and loss of
consciousness.

Clinical picture
In venous air embolism, there is cyanosis, hypotension, syncope and
sometimes death. There is also a characteristic precordial millwheel
murmur.

Management
In venous air embolism clamp the administration set, place the patient in
head down position on his left side so that air remains away from the
pulmonary circulation. If necessary, provide cardiovascular supportive
measures. Large air emboli may be aspirated from the right atrium using
a right atrial catheter.

PHLEBITIS

Pathological physiology
An inflammatory reaction in the vein used for transfusion is common. Its
frequency increases when:
   1. the duration of transfusion (infusion) exceeds 48 hours. New
      sites should be selected every 48 hours and in patients with
      neutropenia or immunosuppression, the sites should be
      changed more often;
   2. long plastic catheters are used; they are more irritant than
      short steel needles;
   3. veins in the lower limbs are used. They are more likely to
      show an inflammatory reaction than the veins in the arms.
      Veins in the lower limbs should only be used exceptionally;

4. small veins are used, since they are more likely to leak and be damaged than large veins. In adults a vein accommodating size 16 catheter should be used whenever possible;
5. irritant intravenous solutions (cytotoxic drugs, antibiotics) are infused. They may even cause permanent vein damage;
6. septic phlebitis is the result of the entry of microorganisms along the venepuncture site. The organisms commonly implicated are *staphylococci* and *corynebacteria*.

Clinical picture

Mild swelling and slight erythema at the site of infusion or along the catheter are common. Marked swelling, erythema along the length of the vein, tenderness, throbbing pain, enlarged local lymph nodes and systemic symptoms of bacteraemia are rare manifestations.

Diagnosis is made clinically. For bacteriological diagnosis send the tip of the catheter in the culture medium, or rinse the needle (removed from the inflamed site) with a small amount of sterile saline or with culture broth, and send this fluid for bacteriological diagnosis.

Management and prevention

Mild phlebitis requires only analgesia and topical warm compresses. In more severe cases appropriate antibiotics should be started. In immunosuppressed or neutropenic patients start treatment with antibiotics (flucloxacillin or erythromycin) as soon as bacteriological material has been collected. Change the antibiotic, if necessary, when the sensitivities are known. In rare instances suppurative phlebitis is so severe that the vein must be surgically ligated at a proximal site and then drained.

Prevention of phlebitis demands strict sterility while inserting the needle or the catheter, or changing infusions and giving treatment. Frequent changes of the transfusion site are also essential. In patients who require long term support with blood, intravenous nutrition or chemotherapy, long central venous or right atrial catheters are recommended. Such catheters (i.e. Hickman's or Broviac) are inserted peripherally using aseptic techniques, and the exit site is fashioned through a subcutaneous tunnel. With meticulous care and frequent changes of sterile dressing, the catheters can remain in site for months without any signs of infection.

REFERENCES

Barton J C 1981 Nonhemolytic, noninfectious transfusion reactions. In: Conrad M E (ed) Transfusion problems in hematology. Seminars in Hematology 18: 95–121
Clement A J 1978 Cardiac and circulatory complications. In: Churchill-Davidson H C (ed) A practice of anaesthesia, 4th edn. Lloyd-Luke Ltd, London, ch 17, p 637–653
Mollison P L 1983 Blood transfusion in clinical medicine, 7th edn. Blackwell Scientific, Oxford
Petz L D, Swisher S N (eds) 1981 Clinical practice of blood transfusion. Churchill Livingstone, Edinburgh

12. DISEASES TRANSMITTED BY TRANSFUSION OF BLOOD AND BLOOD PRODUCTS

One of the serious complications of transfusion of blood and blood products is the transmission of infection. The most frequently transmitted infection is hepatitis (post-transfusion hepatitis, PTH*), caused by hepatitis B virus, or by the virus(es) of non-A, non-B hepatitis. Many other diseases can be transmitted by transfusion, but, with the exception of endemic malaria and Chagas disease, the transmission occurs in isolated cases only.

POST-TRANSFUSION HEPATITIS

Definition of post-transfusion hepatitis embraces all types of infectious hepatitis transmitted by transfusion of blood and blood products. The diagnosis of PTH can be established only after excluding all other modes of transmission, as well as non-infectious causes of hepatic damage.

The incidence of PTH, estimated in prospective studies, is between 1 and 2% for recipients of blood in Europe and Australia, and slightly higher in the USA. The estimated incidence of PTH among recipients of factor VIII concentrate is almost 100%. About 90% of all cases of PTH have a subclinical course.

Etiology
One out of ten cases of PTH is caused by hepatitis B virus (HBV) and of the remainder the majority are due to non-A, non-B hepatitis. Rarely, PTH is caused by other viruses (Table 12.1).

Table 12.1 Viral infections causing post-transfusion hepatitis

Viral infections	Incidence (%)
Hepatitis B*	10
Non-A, non-B hepatitis	90
Hepatitis A	rare
Cytomegalovirus infection	rare
Infection with Epstein-Barr virus	rare

* Testing for hepatitis B virus is mandatory in many countries.

* Post-transfusion hepatitis is the term used by convention. The Council of Europe has recommended the term 'transfusion associated hepatitis' (TAH).

A glossary of terms related to PTH is presented in Table 12.2.

Table 12.2 Glossary of terms relating to post-transfusion hepatitis

Term	Abbreviation
Post-transfusion hepatitis	PTH
(or transfusion associated hepatitis)	(TAH)
Hepatitis B virus	HBV
Hepatitis B surface antigen	HBsAg
Hepatitis B core antigen	HBcAg
Hepatitis B e antigen	HBeAg
Antibody to HBs Ag	Anti-HBs
Antibody to HBc Ag	Anti-HBc
Antibody to HBe Ag	Anti-HBe
Hepatitis non-A, non-B virus(es)	Hepatitis NANB virus(es)
Hepatitis A virus	HAV
Hepatitis A antigen	HAAg
Antibody to HAAg*	Anti-HA
Cytomegalovirus	CMV
Antibody to CMV*	Anti-CMV
Epstein-Barr virus	EBV
Antibody to EBV	Anti-EBV

* Antibody may be of the IgM or IgG class of immunoglobulins.

Hepatitis B

Hepatitis is caused by HBV. The virus, called the Dane particle, consists of double stranded DNA, DNA polymerase and core substance, all enclosed by the viral envelope. Serological markers of HBV are hepatitis B surface antigen (HBsAg), core antigen (HBcAg) and e antigen (HBeAg) which is probably a part of the core. Serological markers of past infection with HBV are antibodies to HBsAg (anti-HBs) and HBcAg (anti-HBc).

Transmission

In addition to transmission by transfusion of blood and blood products the transmission is by:

1. Using blood-contaminated needles for injections, tattooing, ear piercing, hair electrolysis and acupuncture;
2. Sexual contact;
3. Prenatal or perinatal transmission from mothers, who are carriers of HBsAg, to their babies.

Incubation is between six weeks and six months.

Clinical presentation

Malaise, chills and headache are frequent in the prodromal stage. Anorexia and distaste for cigarettes are common early symptoms and nausea, upper abdominal pain and diarrhoea may follow. The liver is tender; splenomegaly and enlarged lymph nodes may occur, particularly in children. Jaundice, pale stools and dark urine are seen in one fifth of the patients. The recovery starts with improved appetite and occurs over a period of three to six weeks. The disease may run a mild course with malaise and vague gastrointestinal complaints as the only symptoms.

The diagnosis is established on the basis of clinical presentation and

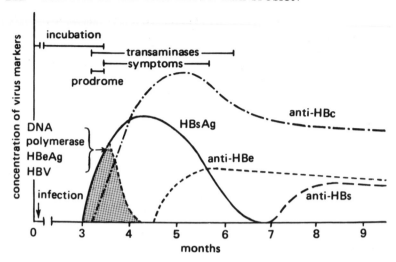

Fig. 12.1 The development of serological markers for hepatitis B in acute HBV infections. (Reproduced from: Tedder R. 1980, with kind permission of the author and editor of the British Journal of Hospital Medicine)

biochemical evidence of hepatitis, and it is confirmed by the detection of markers of HBV (Fig. 12.1). PTH inquiry should be initiated for every patient who has received blood or blood products within six months prior to presenting with hepatitis B.

The treatment is symptomatic.

Prognosis. The majority of patients with hepatitis B recover completely. In the U.K. about 5% of patients become carriers of HBsAg, and about 10% of patients develop chronic hepatitis, which after a number of years may give rise to carcinoma of the liver. Fulminant hepatitis with a fatal outcome occurs in less than 1% of patients.

Carrier state. Carriers are individuals in whom the presence of HBsAg in the circulation has persisted following resolution of an acute infection. Carriers who have demonstrable HBeAg in the plasma in addition to HBsAg are considered more infectious than those who lack HBeAg or have anti-HBe.

Prevention

Testing of blood donors for HBsAg is mandatory in the U.K. and many other countries. Prevention of infection with HBV of individuals at risk, using specific immunoglobulin and a vaccine against HBV is summarised elsewhere (Zuckerman, 1984).

Non-A, Non-B hepatitis

Non-A, non-B hepatitis is probably caused by at least two distinct viruses which are as yet unidentified.

Transmission by transfusion of blood and blood products is well documented. Other yet unidentified modes of transmission must exist, since non-A, non-B hepatitis occurs sporadically in the population.

Incubation is from two weeks to four months. The length of incubation shows a bimodal distribution with two peaks, at two and three months.

Clinical presentation is similar to that seen in hepatitis B, but the disease is milder. Most patients are asymptomatic, and only increased concentrations of serum alanine transferase (ALT), aspartate transferase (AST) and gamma-glutamyl transpeptidase (GGTP) indicate the presence of hepatitis. One fifth of the patients become jaundiced one to four weeks after increased concentrations of transferases in the serum are detected.

The diagnosis is established by exclusion of other causes of hepatitis.

The treatment is symptomatic.

Prognosis. In the majority of patients there is a complete resolution of the disease. In a small proportion of patients chronic hepatitis develops and raised concentrations of ALT and AST in the serum may remain for several years.

A carrier state is likely and may or may not be associated with raised concentrations of serum ALT, AST and GGTP.

Other viruses causing PTH

Hepatitis A

Hepatitis A is caused by hepatitis A virus (HAV). HAV is a single stranded RNA enterovirus.

Transmission is by the fecal-oral route and, exceptionally rarely, by blood collected from donors with viraemia in the prodromal stage of the disease.

Incubation is from 15 to 45 days with a median of 28 days.

Clinical presentation is similar to that of hepatitis B.

The diagnosis is made on the basis of clinical presentation and laboratory findings and is confirmed by detecting antibodies to HAV in the serum, which are initially IgM and later IgG immunoglobulins.

The prognosis is good since the recovery is complete, and the development of chronic liver disease is extremely rare. Carrier status has not been found.

Prevention for the recipient of blood transfusion is not necessary. For use of passive immunisation with normal immunoglobulin and active immunisation with attenuated live virus vaccine see p. 74.

Cytomegalovirus post-transfusion hepatitis

Post-transfusion hepatitis caused by cytomegalovirus (CMV) occurs rarely and almost exclusively in patients who had received massive blood transfusion or who have been immunosuppressed.

The clinical presentation is in the form of 'post-transfusion syndrome' (see below). The disease is mild and its course usually uneventful.

The diagnosis is established on the basis of the clinical presentation, raised concentration of serum ALT and AST, and a rising titre of antibody to CMV. The diagnosis of hepatitis due to CMV should be considered in every case of PTH inquiry. The transmission of CMV infection by blood and its consequences are presented in detail on p. 115.

Hepatitis caused by Epstein-Barr virus (EBV)
This is very rare. The clinical presentation is similar to that of CMV hepatitis and has a mild course. The diagnosis is made by demonstrating heterophile antibody and antibodies to EBV in the serum. The presence of IgM anti-EBV indicates a recent or current infection with EBV. The clinical significance of infection with EBV relates only to the differential diagnosis of post-transfusion hepatitis.

Investigation of post-transfusion hepatitis

The recognition and investigation of PTH occurring in the recipient of blood and blood products is important not only for the management of the patient but also for the identification of the infectious donor. A flow-chart for the investigation of PTH is given in Table 12.3 and the interpretation of serological markers of viral hepatitis is given in Table 12.4.

Table 12.3 Flow chart for investigation of post-transfusion hepatitis

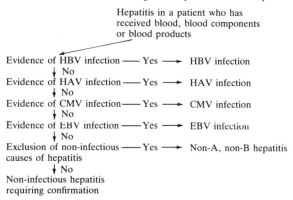

The tracing of the infectious donor is possible only when the unique identification number of each unit of blood and of blood components or batch number of each blood product administered to the patient are recorded.

Prevention of post-transfusion hepatitis

Preventing PTH in recipients of blood and blood products depends, firstly, on strict adherence to the recommendations for the selection of blood donors, and secondly, on rigorous testing for HBsAg carried out

Table 12.4 Interpretation of serological markers of hepatitis B

Clinical interpretation	HbsAg	HbeAg	Anti-HBs	Anti-HBc	Anti-HBe
			Serological marker		
Incubation period	+	+	—	—	—
Acute HB	+	+	—	+	—
Chronic HB	+	+ or —	+ or —	+	+ or —
Carrier state 'e positive'*	+	+	—	+	—
Carrier state 'e negative'	+	—	—	+	+ or —
Infection with HBV without detectable HBsAg	—	—	—	+	—
Past infection with HBV	—	—	+	+	—

* Carriers who are 'e positive' are considerably more infectious than those who are 'e negative'.
For abbreviations see Table 12.2

by the blood collecting centres. However, there is no specific test for detecting non-A, non-B hepatitis. At present it does not seem appropriate to use autotransfusion or collection of blood from the patient's family and friends solely for the purpose of avoiding the risk of PTH.

CYTOMEGALOVIRUS INFECTION TRANSMITTED BY BLOOD TRANSFUSION

Cytomegalovirus (CMV) is one of the herpes viruses, which causes an asymptomatic infection in the majority of infected individuals. CMV is characterised by latency which is probably maintained by the incorporation of genome into the white blood cells, and by activation of infection at the time of reinfection or profound suppression of the host's immune system. CMV is widely spread in the population and evidence of a past infection can be found in about 50% of adults in the Western countries, and in virtually all adults in Africa. In a small number of patients the infection with CMV is a severe and even fatal disease (see below).

Transmission
In addition to being transmitted by blood, and in particular by platelet and granulocyte concentrates, CMV is transmitted by:
  1. intrauterine or perinatal infection and by breast feeding in neonates and infants;
  2. close contact in children;
  3. probably by kissing and sexual contact in young adults.
  Incubation in primary infection is between three weeks and four months with a median of four weeks. In reinfection or reactivation with the latent virus, laboratory diagnostic tests become positive after an incubation period from one to 18 months, with a median of seven months.

Clinical presentation
  1. *Neonates*. Over 90% of infections are asymptomatic, about 5 to 10% of infections are mild with transient jaundice and

purpura, mild hepatosplenomegaly and failure to thrive, and less than 1% have cytomegalic inclusion disease, which presents with hepatosplenomegaly, haemorrhagic diathesis and interstitial pneumonia. A late consequence of infection with CMV is mental retardation, found in a small proportion of cases, including some of those who have had an inapparent infection.

2. *Adults* have either an asymptomatic infection or the 'CMV mononucleosis syndrome' with fever, lymphadenopathy, hepatosplenomegaly, rarely jaundice and the presence of atypical lymphocytes in the peripheral blood. *Patients* following massive transfusion of blood may present with a similar, 'post-transfusion syndrome' caused either by primary infection or reactivation of the latent virus.

3. *Recipients of renal transplants* The incidence of CMV in patients with renal transplants is about 40%. Primary infection presents with fever, epigastric pain, hepatosplenomegaly, abnormal liver function tests, leucopenia, thrombocytopenia and atypical mononuclear cells in the peripheral blood film, and pulmonary infiltration on chest X-ray. Reactivation is associated with a mild form of the disease, usually without fever and hepatosplenomegaly. CMV infection may adversely affect the function of the graft and in a small proportion of patients may contribute to graft failure.

4. *Recipients of bone marrow transplants* are also affected by primary infection or reinfection with CMV. The incidence of infection is about 50%. The clinical presentation is similar to that seen in patients with renal transplants. Patients receiving granulocyte transfusions are particularly at risk from CMV infection. CMV pneumonitis, which occurs in about 16% of patients, is a serious and often fatal complication of marrow transplantation and represents the highest single cause of death in transplanted patients.

The diagnosis of a past infection can be conveniently established using radioimmunoassay, complement fixation assay or indirect haemagglutination test for antibody to CMV. Detection of IgM anti-CMV indicates recent infection.

The treatment of severe infection with CMV has not been very successful. It consists of:

1. reduction of immunosuppressive treatment (in patients with renal transplants);
2. antiviral chemotherapy, for example acyclovir (5 mg/kg body weight/8 hours, i.v.);
3. administration of anti-CMV immunoglobulin or plasma with a high titre of antibody to CMV.

Prevention is considered only for patients who are likely to suffer from serious consequences of CMV infection:
1. premature and low birth weight babies;
2. patients with renal transplants;
3. patients with bone marrow transplants.

Preventive measures aimed at pregnant women who are found negative on testing for anti-CMV do not seem to be justified. At present the mainstay of prevention is transfusion of blood and blood components collected from donors who are found negative on testing for anti-CMV. Passive immunisation with anti-CMV immunoglobulin is available and active immunisation using vaccines is currently under investigation.

ACQUIRED IMMUNE DEFICIENCY SYNDROME ASSOCIATED WITH TRANSFUSION

Definition
Acquired immunodeficiency syndrome (AIDS), as defined by the Center for Disease Control (Atlanta, Georgia, USA), includes reliably diagnosed diseases indicative of underlying cellular immunodeficiency in the absence of any other cause of reduced resistance or increased susceptibility to that disease. These diseases include opportunistic infections such as *Pneumocystis carinii*, Kaposi's sarcoma in persons under 60 years of age and lymphoma limited to the brain. The causative agent of AIDS is presumed to be a retrovirus, called human T-cell lymphotropic virus type III (HTLV III) by the American authors, or lymphadenopathy-associated virus (LAV) by the French authors.

Incidence
Just over 10 000 cases of AIDS have been recognised world-wide and of that number in about 1% evidence suggests that the disease was acquired by transfusion of blood or blood products. The majority of the cases have been described in the U.S.A. and only a small proportion has been found in Europe or in individuals who have lived in Central Africa where HTLV III may be endemic.

Transmission
Epidemiological evidence suggests that the HTLV III can be transmitted in several ways:
1. by administration of factor VIII concentrates to persons with haemophilia and probably of blood and blood products to other persons;
2. by sexual contact between homosexual men as well as from bisexual and heterosexual men to their female partners; this mode of transmission is the most frequent;
3. by sharing contaminated needles between drug addicts; and
4. by intrauterine infection in babies born to infected mothers.

Table 12.5 Epidemiology of AIDS and frequency of cases in the major at-risk groups

At-risk groups	Per cent of total number of cases
Homosexual or bisexual males	71
Intravenous drug abusers	17
Haitians	5
Haemophiliacs/blood transfusion recipients	1
Female partners of patients with AIDS	
Children of mothers with AIDS	6
Patients with AIDS who do not belong to an at-risk group	

Modified from: Pinching, 1984

'At risk' groups

The epidemiology indicates that patients with AIDS belong to several 'at risk' groups (Table 12.5). Patients receiving blood and blood products are at a very low risk of acquiring AIDS when the risk is measured against the total number of units of blood administered. However, a substantial proportion of haemophiliacs who received large doses of factor VIII concentrate in the past are positive when tested for anti-HTLV III (see below).

Incubation is long, probably between one and three years or longer.

Clinical presentation, which reflects the degree of reduction in numbers of T_4 lymphocytes, the target cells for HTLV III, may be preceded by malaise and appearance of swollen lymph nodes, intermittent fever, and in some instances night sweats, diarrhoea and weight loss (pre-AIDS or lymphoadenopathy syndrome). The commonest presenting features are (i) opportunistic infections, in particular infection with *Pneumocystis carinii* with rapidly progressive interstitial pneumonitis, *Candida, Pseudomonas, Staphylococcus* and *Enterobacteriaceae*, (ii) Kaposi's sarcoma or various types of non-Hodgkin's lymphoma, and (iii) simultaneous development of infections and tumours.

The diagnosis is based on clinical presentation, detection of antibodies to HTLV III (anti-HTLV III) in the serum as well as by demonstrating immunosuppression in a person from one of the 'at risk' groups. There is cutaneous anergy, decreased in vitro lymphocytic response to stimulation, decreased number of T lymphocytes, decreased ratio of T helper and T suppressor lymphocytes, decreased number of natural killer cells, increased concentration of serum gamma globulins and increased activity of B lymphocytes. The significance of a positive anti-HTLV III test in an otherwise healthy person is not yet clear.

Treatment is symptomatic.

The prognosis is grave since no patient has been shown to recover cellular immunity, and the overall mortality is about 50%, increasing proportionally with the length of time since diagnosis.

Prevention of transfusion transmitted AIDS has been based so far on voluntary self-exclusion of donors in the 'at risk' groups from donating blood. Testing blood donations for anti-HTLV III is expected to be introduced in the UK soon.

SYPHILIS FOLLOWING BLOOD TRANSFUSION

Syphilis is a systemic and chronic infectious disease, caused by *Treponema pallidum* and characterised by florid manifestations and long periods of quiescence. Its occurrence following blood transfusion is exceptionally rare.

Transmission is usually by sexual contact, and very rarely by a non-sexual route as in congenital and endemic syphilis, by sharing contaminated needles among drug addicts and by blood transfusion.

Incubation is between two and four weeks for sexually transmitted disease, but eight to 12 weeks following blood transfusion.

Clinical presentation. When the infection is transmitted by blood the typical local lesion (chancre) of *primary syphilis* does not occur and the disease presents as *secondary syphilis*. Symptoms are malaise, headache, fever and general aches and pains. Signs are many and variable; three quarters of the patients have a macular rash on the trunk, limbs, palms and soles, one half have enlarged, discrete, rubbery and non-tender lymph nodes, and one third mucosal ulcers. If the diagnosis is not made at that stage symptoms and signs will gradually disappear even without treatment and the disease will enter its latent form. About 60% of patients who reach the latent stage will remain in that stage without further progression. *Tertiary syphilis* may develop three to ten years or more after the primary infection in the patient who has not been treated earlier. Tertiary syphilis is characterised by the formation of gummas and in a small proportion of patients by manifestations of cardiovascular syphilis and neurosyphilis.

The diagnosis is made by demonstrating *T.pallidum* in the skin and mucosal lesions and by serological testing using the non-specific cardiolipin VDRL test, and the specific tests such as the haemagglutination test (TPHA), the fluorescent treponemal antibody test (FTA) and the treponemal immobilisation test (TPI). These tests cannot be used to differentiate between syphilis and other treponemal diseases (yaws, bejel and pinta).

The treatment of syphilis is with penicillin. Patients with secondary syphilis should receive procain penicillin, 600 mg daily for 15 days or benzathine penicillin, 2.4 megaunits weekly for three weeks. Patients with allergy to penicillin should receive erythromycin or tetracycline, 500 mg six hourly for 15 days.

Prevention. Testing each donation of blood for serological evidence of syphilis is mandatory in the U.K. and many other countries, and donations which yield positive results are not used for transfusion or fractionation of plasma. Treponemae are inactivated in blood after 72 hours at 6°C and in plasma components on freezing below −20°C.

PROTOZOAN INFECTIONS TRANSMITTED BY TRANSFUSION

Malaria

Malaria is an infectious febrile disease produced by several species of plasmodia, *P.vivax, P.falciparun, P.malariae*, and *P.ovale*. Transfusion malaria is encountered in areas where the disease is endemic. Sporadic cases seen in other parts of the world are brought in by travellers from endemic areas.

Transmission by blood transfusion and among drug addicts by syringes contaminated with blood is very rare. Natural transmission is only from host to host by bite of an infected anopheline mosquito.

Incubation is six days for *P.vivax*, 12 days for *P.falciparum* and 18 to 40 days for *P.malariae*.

Clinical presentation. Paroxysms of severe chills, fever and sweating may occur daily (quotidian), on alternate days (tertian) or with an interval of two days (quartan). After recovery from the acute attack the untreated disease has a tendency to become chronic with occasional relapses.

Treatment of malaria caused by *P.falciparum* is with chloroquine unless resistance is suspected. Treatment of malaria caused by *P.vivax, P.malariae* and *P.ovale* is with chloroquine and primaquine. For treatment schedules see medical textbooks.

Prevention of malaria in general is by prophylactic administration of antimalarial drugs. Prevention of transfusion malaria in countries where malaria is not endemic is carried out as part of the procedure for selection of donors. Current recommendations in the U.K. are that blood, collected from donors who have had malaria or who were born or lived in areas with endemic malaria, is used only as plasma for fractionation, and that blood from donors who have visited areas with endemic malaria, is only used for transfusion to patients if the donor has returned to the U.K. at least eight weeks prior to donation, was taking anti-malarial drugs during his stay and for one month after returning, and has had no illness since returning.

Prevention of transfusion malaria in countries with endemic malaria is achieved by administration of chloroquine (base 600 mg i.m.) to each recipient of blood immediately following transfusion.

Chagas' disease

Chagas' disease is caused by *Trypanosoma cruzii*. It is a progressive, non-contagious, insect transmitted disease established in the Central and South Americas.

Transmission is by blood-sucking insects. It may be transmitted by transfusion of blood and blood components.

Clinical presentation. The initial lesion usually involves the eye but may be cutaneous; it is unilateral, accompanied by periorbital oedema, regional lymphadenopathy, often enlargement of the lacrimal gland and fever. Symptoms and signs resolve after one to three months. In the acute stage which is frequently associated with the initial lesion, there are intermittent fever, oedema, generalised lymphadenopathy, exanthemata, and nodular subcutaneous lesion (chagomas). With abatement of the acute symptoms the disease may terminate or may be followed by an asymptomatic period which after a variable length of time terminates with major manifestations of chronic Chagas' disease: cardiopathy, mega-oesophagus and mega-colon.

The diagnosis is made by demonstrating *T.cruzii* in the blood, cerebro-spinal fluid or biopsy material; serologically by a complement fixation test, the methylene blue technique (dye test) or with fluorescein-labelled antibody.

Treatment. There is no satisfactory treatment.

Prevention. Prophylactic measures are centred on insect control. Transmission by transfusion is prevented by (i) screening of donors with the dye test and rejection of units with a high titre of antibodies, and (ii) addition of gentian violet, 125 mg, to each unit of blood, to kill the parasites without causing haemolysis or toxicity to the recipient.

Other protozoan infections

Transmission of African trypanosomiasis, kala-azar and toxoplasmosis by blood transfusion has been reported in isolated cases but is of little clinical significance.

BACTERIAL INFECTIONS TRANSMITTED BY TRANSFUSION

Bacteria may find their way into the blood pack either via the blood collected from a donor with transient bacteraemia or by contamination of the pack itself.

Bacteraemia in the donor

A person with significant bacteraemia is unlikely to donate blood. Donors who may have transient bacteraemia following minor dental or surgical procedures as well as those with fever or taking antibiotics are deferred; donors who are long term carriers of pathogenic bacteria are exceptionally rare.

Bacterial contamination of blood and blood components

Contamination of the pack can occur during venepuncture, through pin-holes in the plastic or through leaking seals. Most of the organisms do not survive the bactericidal properties of the anticoagulant, plasma and low temperature. However, species of coliforms (*E.coli, A.aerogenes, Kl.pneumoniae*), pseudomonas and proteus, capable of multiplying in a refrigerator or at room temperature, have been implicated in severe bacterial infections transmitted by transfusion.

Clinical presentation resembles experimental endotoxin shock. Headache, backache, nausea, and abdominal cramps occur within an hour of transfusion. Fever may be high and the blood pressure may fall dramatically.

Management

Stop transfusion immediately and start the procedure for investigating a transfusion reaction described on p. 92. The differential diagnosis is between haemolytic and non-haemolytic transfusion reactions and a reaction due to transfusion of contaminated blood. The presence of bacteria on stained smears and/or growth of bacteria in a culture medium confirms the diagnosis. Treatment is aimed at improving hydration, combating shock with hydrocortisone and volume expanders, and treatment of sepsis using wide spectrum antibiotics.

Prevention

1. Units of blood should be left at room temperature for the shortest possible time, and never longer than 30 min.
2. Processing of blood using 'open' techniques should be performed in a laminar flow cabinet, or preferably in a sterile suit.
3. Each unit of blood or red cells should be carefully inspected for haemolysis immediately before transfusion.

Note that granulocyte and platelet concentrates are kept at room temperature for one and up to five days, respectively. There has been no evidence of increased incidence of bacterial contamination among concentrates on sterility testing.

REFERENCES

Adler M W 1984 Syphilis: clinical features. British Medical Journal 288: 468–471
Adler M W 1984 Syphilis: diagnosis and management. British Medical Journal 288: 551–553
Barbara J A J 1983 Microbiology in blood transfusion. Wright, Bristol
Bayer W L, Tegtmeier G E, Barbara J A J 1984 The significance of non-A, non-B hepatitis, cytomegalovirus and the acquired immune deficiency syndrome in transfusion practice. In: Bayer W L (ed) Blood transfusion and blood banking. Clinics in Haematology 13: 254–269
Bruce-Chwatt L J 1982 Transfusion malaria revisited. Tropical Diseases Bulletin 79: 827–840
Conrad M E 1981 Diseases transmissible by blood transfusion: viral hepatitis and other infectious disorders. In: Conrad M E (ed) Transfusion problems in hematology. Seminars in Hematology 18: 122–146
Curran J W, Lawrence D N, Jaffe H et al 1984 Acquired immunodeficiency syndrome (AIDS) associated with transfusions. New England Journal of Medicine 310: 69–75
Pinching A J 1984 Acquired immune deficiency syndrome. Hospital Update 10: 117–129
Tedder R 1980 Hepatitis B in hospitals. British Journal of Hospital Medicine 23: 266–279
Zuckerman A J 1984 Who should be immunised against hepatitis B? British Medical Journal 289: 1243–1244

13. CLINICAL SYNDROMES OF FETO-MATERNAL INCOMPATIBILITY

Feto-maternal incompatibility is a term used to describe clinical syndromes in the fetus caused by the placental transfer of a maternal alloantibody (Table 13.1).

Table 13.1 Clinical syndromes of feto-maternal incompatibility

Syndrome	Target cells	System of cell antigens involved
Haemolytic disease of the newborn	red blood cells	ABO, Rhesus, Kell, Duffy and other
Alloimmune neonatal thrombocytopenia	platelets	Pl^{A1} and other
Alloimmune neonatal neutropenia	granulocytes	NA, HLA

HAEMOLYTIC DISEASE OF THE NEWBORN

The most frequently encountered syndrome is the haemolytic disease of the newborn (HDN). In HDN the fetal red cell life span is shortened due to destruction by maternal alloantibody. The antibody is directed to an antigen of the ABO or Rh systems or, in rare instances, to an antigen of other blood group systems (Kell, Duffy, Kidd, MNSs, etc.). HDN due to Rh incompatibility is clinically much more important than ABO incompatibility although it is estimated that the latter occurs much more frequently.

The severity of HDN varies widely: when haemolysis is mild it can be detected only by laboratory testing; severe HDN, however, carries a high risk of stillbirth and perinatal death. The management of HDN is complex and requires the combined skills of the obstetrician, radiologist, paediatrician and haematologist (with an interest in blood transfusion) as well as the general practitioner and primary care team. As the incidence of severe HDN has been significantly reduced since the introduction of routine administration of anti-D immunoglobulin at delivery for prevention of Rh alloimmunisation following pregnancy, few hospitals have retained the necessary skills to manage severe cases of HDN, and the most rewarding results are now being achieved in specialised centres.

HAEMOLYTIC DISEASE OF THE NEWBORN DUE TO ANTI-Rh

Definition
Haemolysis of Rh(D)-positive fetal red cells by maternal anti-D* antibody.

Incidence of Rh HDN in a given population is proportional to the prevalence of the Rh(D)-negative phenotype. The incidence of that phenotype is 15% in the British population, but it varies from 0% in Japanese, Chinese and American Indians to 20% in some European countries. Before the routine use of anti-D immunoglobulin for prevention of HDN was introduced, 60 to 70 cases of HDN per 10 000 births were found in a white population. This figure is fifteen times lower than expected on theoretical grounds because of the following:

1. sensitisation to Rh(D) antigen usually does not occur in the first pregnancy;
2. half of the babies from Rh(D) heterozygous fathers are Rh(D) negative;
3. only one out of eight Rh(D)-negative women bearing a Rh(D) positive child develops anti-D antibodies.

Since the routine use of anti-D immunoglobulin for the prevention of HDN was introduced the incidence of HDN has fallen more than ten times. However, the morbidity and perinatal mortality associated with HDN remain high: about 40% of neonates with HDN require no treatment, 20% require only phototherapy for hyperbilirubinaemia, 20% require one or more exchange transfusions and 20% require intrauterine transfusions and/or other special measures. The mortality of HDN is at present about one in 10 000 live births.

Pathogenesis

Immunisation of the mother

Immunisation by pregnancy
In most normal pregnancies small numbers of fetal red cells enter the maternal circulation late in pregnancy or at delivery. The likelihood of immunisation after a feto-maternal bleed increases with the size of the bleed and is greater when it occurs early in pregnancy. In toxaemia, in the presence of placental abnormalities, during external rotation or manual removal of the placenta, larger numbers of fetal red cells may enter the maternal circulation. In one out of 50 pregnancies a feto-maternal bleed takes place early in the pregnancy and in about one out of 200 pregnancies the 'bleed' is greater than 10 ml of fetal red cells. Anti-D antibody appears in the mother's circulation six weeks to six

---

* In rare instances other Rh antibodies, anti-c, –E and –C, may cause HDN, which is usually mild.

months after the feto-maternal bleed and in some women the antibody becomes detectable only after the second exposure to D antigen.

Immunisation by transfusion of blood or blood products
Administration of 200 ml of Rh(D)-positive red cells, contained in a unit of blood, will immunise two out of three Rh(D)-negative recipients. Therefore, in cases of inadvertent administration of Rh(D)-positive blood to a Rh(D)-negative woman of childbearing age an attempt to prevent immunisation must be made (p. 77).

Leucocyte concentrates and *buffy coats* contain substantial numbers of red cells and the guidelines for the selection of the Rh group are the same as for red cells (p. 59). Since *platelet concentrates* contain only a very small number of red cells, Rh(D)-positive platelets may be transfused to Rh(D)-negative recipients when Rh(D)-negative platelets are not available, but women of childbearing age should be protected from immunisation by intramuscular administration of 100 μg (500 i.u.) of anti-D immunoglobulin (p. 77). At present there is no evidence that *fresh frozen plasma* or *cryoprecipitate*, prepared from Rh(D)-positive units of blood, cause primary immunisation when administered to Rh(D)-negative recipients.

The effect of maternal anti-D on the fetus
In HDN the maternal IgG anti-D alloantibody crosses the placenta and coats the fetal red cells which are then destroyed by the mononuclear macrophage system in the spleen. The rate of haemolysis depends on the avidity of the antibody and its concentration in the fetal circulation. The main consequence of haemolysis is anaemia. Chronic anaemia leads to massive erythroid hyperplasia in the liver and spleen, causing hepatosplenomegaly. Profound anaemia may cause oedema, ascites and anasarca (hydrops fetalis), as well as cardiac failure leading to death in utero. The high rate of bilirubin production is almost matched by the rate of clearance via the placenta and the fetus is not in danger of hyperbilirubinaemia. HDN in the first affected pregnancy is usually milder than that in the second and subsequent pregnancies.

HDN in the neonate
At the time of birth the placental transfer of anti-D ceases and the rate of haemolysis gradually abates over a period of weeks. However, the clearance of bilirubin by the placenta also ceases and the capacity of the liver to conjugate bilirubin in the neonate is exceeded. Consequently the bilirubin concentration increases rapidly; thus the main feature of HDN is a rapid development of jaundice (icterus praecox). HDN may be graded as mild, moderate or severe by the clinical presentation and the concentration of haemoglobin and bilirubin.

Mild HDN
The haemoglobin concentration in the cord blood is within the normal range for neonates or only slightly reduced and the bilirubin concentration rises within the first day of life but at no time exceeds 75 μmol/l. No treatment is required.

Moderate HDN presents with rapidly increasing bilirubin concentration (icterus praecox) and usually mild anaemia. The rise of bilirubin concentration must be halted by exchange transfusion to protect the CNS from the toxic effects of bilirubin. Deposition of bilirubin in the CNS causes permanent neurological damage (ataxia, mental retardation, deafness) and it is termed 'kernicterus' because of icteric staining of the basal ganglia and cerebellum.

Severe HDN presents with profound anaemia, oedema, cardiac failure, tissue hypoxia and acidosis. Hypoalbuminaemia may also be present contributing to oedema and deposition of bilirubin in the tissues. Profound anaemia may cause death in utero from about the eighteenth week of gestation onwards. At birth the infant suffers from the consequences of both anaemia and hyperbilirubinaemia.

It must be remembered that the consequences of HDN are more pronounced in premature and low birth weight infants.

Antenatal investigation and management

At the time of the first visit to the antenatal clinic every pregnant woman should give a detailed obstetric history and provide a sample of blood for blood group determination and antibody screen. In the absence of history of HDN the antibody screen should be repeated at 28 and 36 weeks of gestation (Table 13.2).

When an antibody is detected in the serum of a pregnant woman, it should be identified and measured, and a follow-up should be arranged in two to three weeks time. Whenever possible a sample of blood from the father should be obtained and his blood group and phenotype determined. Further managment will depend on the type of antibody, its initial concentration in the serum and the rise of its concentration on the next and subsequent follow-ups. When the concentration of anti-D is less than 4 i.u./ml (0.8 µg/ml, approximate titre 1:16) and when there is no change in its concentration, the measurement should be repeated at two to three week intervals.

Amniocentesis is indicated when the concentration of anti-D is higher than 4 i.u./ml (0.8 µg/ml; titre 1:16) or when it has risen since the last determination. Amniocentesis is usually carried out after the 18th week of gestation and provides information on the severity of HDN and the maturity of the fetus. When it is carried out using a fetoscope a sample of fetal blood can be obtained for the determination of phenotype and concentrations of haemoglobin and bilirubin. Since the concentration of bilirubin in the amniotic fluid is proportional to that in the plasma it is possible to estimate the severity of HDN by plotting values for optical density due to bilirubin in the amniotic fluid on a Liley's chart (Fig. 13.1 and 13.2). The position of the initial value on the chart and the trend in subsequent measurements, will determine further action:

    1. When the initial value is in zone 3 and repeated measurements reveal no upward trend the baby is either

Table 13.2 Management flow-chart for Rh(D) negative women during pregnancy

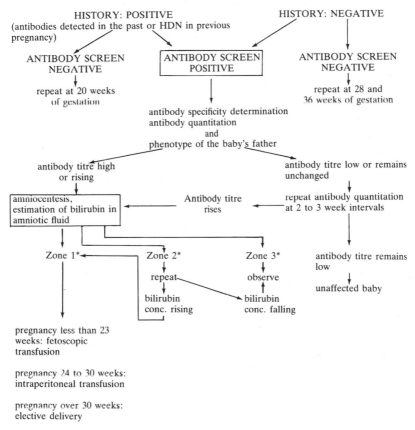

* See Fig. 13.2

Rh(D)-negative or only mildly affected, and no action is required.

2. When the initial value is in zone 2 amniocentesis should be repeated within two to three weeks to establish the trend.

3. When the initial value is in zone 1 the baby is severely affected and in danger of imminent death. The management entails intrauterine transfusions until it becomes possible to perform elective delivery.

Intrauterine transfusion maintains the haemoglobin concentration of a severely affected baby until it reaches sufficient maturity to be delivered.

Blood required. Group O Rh(D) negative, less than 48 hours old, concentrated or washed red cells with haematocrit of 0.80 to 0.90 l/l. When the fetal blood group is known group specific red cells are transfused. Whenever possible blood negative on testing for anti-CMV antibody should be used.

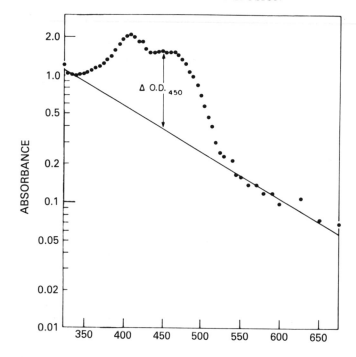

Fig. 13.1 Visible absorption spectrum of amniotic fluid. Absorbency is plotted against wavelength. The line connecting the beginning and the tail of the absorption curve represents background absorbency. The height of the peak at 450 nm (Δ OD 450) is directly related to the severity of the disease of the fetus in utero. (Reproduced form *Technical Manual of the American Association of Blood Banks*, 8th edn, with kind permission of the American Association of Blood Banks)

Procedure
The volume of blood used for administration *into the intraperitoneal cavity* depends on the gestational age and varies from 40 ml at 24 weeks to 100 ml at 30 weeks. Transfusions may be repeated at two to three week intervals. Transfusion *into the umbilical cord vessels* using a fetoscope has been recently introduced. Under direct vision a transfusion can be given earlier in the course of pregnancy. About 15 ml of blood is injected. Blood can be also withdrawn from the cord and it is possible to exchange 5 ml aliquots of blood several times.

Fetal death due to amniocentesis is very rare, but if blood sampling is attempted at the same time, the incidence of fetal death is about 5%. Of babies undergoing intrauterine transfusions about half survive, and of these up to 4% have some major disability resulting from the disease or its treatment. Perinatal mortality is about 20% when elective delivery at 28 weeks of pregnancy is carried out, but it is substantially lower when it is carried out after the 30th week.

Elective delivery can be performed from the 28th week of gestation in

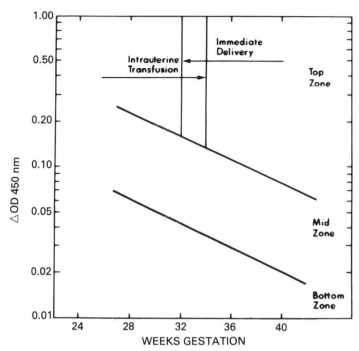

Fig. 13.2 Modified Liley graph used for interpretation of data from amniotic fluid studies. Top zone is zone 1 in the text, mid zone is zone 2 and bottom zone is zone 3. An intrauterine transfusion should be done if the OD value is in the top zone prior to 32 weeks gestation. After 34 weeks values in the top zone indicate immedate delivery. Either may be indicated between 32 and 34 weeks, depending on the fetal maturity. (Reproduced from *Technical Manual of the American Association of Blood Banks*, 8th edn, with kind permission of the American Association of Blood Banks)

centres having neonatal intensive care units. Elective delivery is routinely performed from the 30th week of gestation when there is evidence of severe HDN (the value of optical density of the amniotic fluid due to bilirubin is in zone 1) and when there is a high sphyngomyelin/lecithin ratio in the amniotic fluid indicating lung maturity.

Planning the investigation and management

The choice and timing of invasive investigative procedures should be made according to the circumstances of each individual case. Amniocentesis will invalidate results obtained by quantitation of anti-D in the mother's circulation. Following an intrauterine transfusion the measurement of optical density of the amniotic fluid will no longer provide reliable information on the baby's condition; determination of bilirubin in the baby's blood samples by fetoscopy would then be required instead. Alternatively one can use ultrasound for measuring the baby's abdominal circumference; the increase of the latter is a poor prognostic sign.

Plasma exchange

The role of plasma exchange for removing anti-D from the maternal circulation is as yet undecided. It is generally accepted that the concentration of anti-D higher than 4 i.u./ml is a valid indication for plasma exchange. However, there is little agreement on the validity of other indications for plasma exchange, and therefore, each patient should be assessed on her own merit. A decision to undertake a programme of plasma exchanges should be made early in pregnancy, or even before conception in a planned pregnancy, so that exchanges can start between the eighth and tenth week of gestation. Plasma exchange is carried out once or twice weekly and 2 to 4 l of plasma are exchanged each time, although good responses have been claimed with exchanges of only 0.5 l per week.

Some problems of antenatal investigation

Women who attend the antenatal clinic for the first time late in pregnancy and are found to have a high concentration of anti-D require amniocentesis for the assessment of the severity of HDN.

Each pregnancy in a Rh(D)-negative woman who possesses anti-D should be regarded as at risk regardless of the father's phenotype, until it is proven that the fetus is not affected by HDN.

All pregnant women, whether Rh(D) negative or positive, should be screened for the presence of antibodies, so that antibodies against one of the Rh antigens other than D, or antigens outside the Rh system can be detected.

HDN in the neonate

Clinical presentation

Babies born with *severe HDN* have low APGAR scores, they are anaemic, hypoxic, acidotic, in cardiac failure, with raised peripheral venous pressure, and oedema, and may have clinical signs of disseminated intravascular coagulation. Such babies may die within a few hours of birth despite resuscitation. In *moderately severe HDN* the most striking finding is the rapid development of jaundice and rise of serum bilirubin concentration. Often clinical signs of anaemia are absent. *Mild HDN* is detected by laboratory investigation only.

Table 13.3 Findings in cord blood from HDN cases of varying severity

Severity of HDN	TESTS		
	Haemoglobin concentration (g/dl)	Reticulocytes (%)	Serum bilirubin concentration (μmol/l)
Severe	<10.5	>20*	>150
Moderate	10 to 13**	10 to 20	>70
Mild	>13**	7 to 10	>20

* Many nucleated red cells are present on the film.
** Some authorities extend the range of anaemia to 14 g/dl.

Laboratory investigations
Initially, haemoglobin concentration, PCV, white cell count, platelet count, reticulocyte count, DIC screen, direct antiglobulin test and serum bilirubin concentration are determined. The pattern of results in severe, moderate and mild HDN is shown in Table 13.3. Monitoring of the severely affected premature neonate in the intensive therapy unit often requires a battery of tests performed at hourly intervals. Moderately affected babies usually require serial determinations of concentrations of bilirubin and haemoglobin.

Management
The severely affected baby, especially when premature and of low birth weight, will be nursed in an incubator and will likely need intubation, ventilation, treatment for cardiac failure and exchange transfusion (exchange transfusion is described in Chapter 3). Hypoglycaemia, hypocalcaemia and hypoproteinaemia should be corrected when present. Serum bilirubin is monitored at least six hourly and usually more often.
In some cases of severe HDN, a 'rebound hyperbilirubinaemia', that is the unabated rise of bilirubin after exchange transfusion, is caused by equilibration between the extravascular and intravascular bilirubin spaces on the one hand, and continuing haemolysis of the newly produced Rh(D)-positive red cells. Several exchange transfusions may be required before the concentration of bilirubin is lowered to a safe level.

In the moderately affected baby exchange transfusion is used to remove excess bilirubin. The decision to use exchange transfusion rather than phototherapy depends on the maturity of the baby and the rate of rise of the serum bilirubin concentration (Table 13.4) which should be measured at least six hourly.

Table 13.4 Bilirubin concentration and the management of HDN after the baby's birth

| Bilirubin concentration (μmol/l) | Baby's age | | |
	up to 24 hours	24 to 72 hours	over 72 hours
less than 70	observe	—	—
70 to 150	phototherapy	observe	—
over 150*	exchange transfusion	phototherapy	observe

* if bilirubin exceeds 250 μmol/l exchange transfusion is required regardless of baby's age or cause of hyperbilirubinaemia.

Follow-up

The infant
A proportion of babies develop 'late' anaemia. In infants who have not received an exchange transfusion this may be due to continuing mild haemolysis. In those who received an exchange transfusion mild anaemia may be the result of transient marrow suppression or repeat sampling of blood for tests. Small supplementary transfusions ('top-ups') will restore

haemoglobin concentration to the normal value. Rh-negative red cells should be used.

The mother

Anti-D should be measured six months *post partum* in all women in whom anti-D was detected during the pregnancy. If the mother wishes to become pregnant again, it is the best time to discuss the prospects of the next pregnancy, and when appropriate make plans for plasma exchange and offer genetic counselling. Women wishing to have children, who have a poor obstetric history, no living child, and a husband homozygous for Rh(D) antigen may wish to consider artificial insemination by a donor (AID) who is Rh(D) negative.

Prevention of Rh haemolytic disease of the newborn

Prevention of Rh(D) haemolytic disease of the newborn is achieved by administering anti-D immunoglobulin to Rh(D)-negative women following sensitising obstetrical events and delivery, or transfusion with Rh(D)-positive blood and blood components. Anti-D immunoglobulin coats the Rh(D)-positive red cells which leads to their immediate removal from the circulation by the mononuclear phagocyte system. Thus the mechanism of antigen recognition by lymphocytes is bypassed and sensitisation to the Rh(D) antigen prevented. Indications for administration of anti-D immunoglobulin, available preparations, its administration and the monitoring of its effect are outlined below and presented in detail in Chapter 7.

Prevention of sensitisation

It is *advisable* to perform a fetal cell count (the Kleihauer test) on the blood of Rh(D)-negative women to determine the size of any transplacental haemorrhage following delivery, abortion and sensitising events during pregnancy.

It is *essential* that all Rh(D)-negative women receive an appropriate dose of anti-D immunoglobulin after:
1. delivery of an Rh(D)-positive fetus;
2. abortion (spontaneous or therapeutic) at whatever stage of pregnancy this occurs;
3. every sensitising event during pregnancy (i.e. whenever there is a particular risk of transplacental haemorrhage from threatened abortion, antepartum haemorrhage, version, amniocentesis, injuries, etc.).

The *recommended standard dose* of anti-D immunoglobulin, for intramuscular administration, following delivery or abortion at 20 weeks and over is 100 μg (500 i.u.), following abortion up to 20 weeks is 50 μg (250 i.u.), and following any other sensitising episode is 100 μg (500 i.u.). The dose should be augmented when the fetal cell count indicates that the transplacental haemorrhage has exceeded 4 ml of fetal cells (see p. 78). It may be necessary to repeat the fetal cell count following a large transplacental bleed to check that all fetal cells have been eliminated.

The anti-D immunoglobulin should be administered within 72 hours of delivery, abortion or other sensitising episode and preferably within the first 24 hours. However anti-D immunoglobulin should not be withheld if the 72 hour period has been exceeded.

The prevention of sensitisation of Rh(D)-negative women by using anti-D immunoglobulin has reduced the incidence of HDN by at least ten times. In addition, the perinatal mortality due to HDN has been reduced by improved paediatric care. However, the hope of eliminating HDN by preventive measures has not been fulfilled, first, because some women become sensitised before or during the first pregnancy, secondly, because a small number of women fail to receive anti-D immunoglobulin, receive it too late or in inadequate quantity, and thirdly, because there is as yet no prevention of HDN caused by antibodies other than anti-D.

HAEMOLYTIC DISEASE OF THE NEWBORN DUE TO ABO INCOMPATIBILITY

Definition
Haemolysis of fetal red cells brought about by maternal anti-A or anti-B (IgG) alloantibodies. The disease is confined to babies of blood group A or B born to mothers of group O. Exceptionally, a group A_2 mother with anti-A_1 antibody may have a baby of blood group A_1 with HDN.

Incidence
It is estimated that the ABO feto-maternal incompatibility occurs in 15% of all pregnancies, that it can be detected in one out of 25 ABO incompatible pregnancies and that it causes HDN of sufficient severity to require exchange transfusion in only one out of 400 incompatible pregnancies. HDN due to ABO incompatibility is more common in Negroes.

The reasons for the apparent rarity of overt HDN in ABO incompatibility are:

1. only immune (IgG) anti-A and anti-B antibodies cross the placenta;
2. in the newborn, red cells have a smaller number of A or B antigenic sites than in the adult;
3. the reaction between the maternal antibody and fetal red cells may be modified by the presence of A or B substance in the plasma and on the surface of other cells.

Pathogenesis

Fetal red cells are coated by the maternal immune (IgG) anti-A or anti-B and trapped in the spleen or liver. There the coated red cells come into contact with phagocytes and may be destroyed (extravascular haemolysis) or may lose only a part of the membrane before being released into the circulation as spherocytes.

Investigation and management

Clinical presentation
HDN due to ABO incompatibility is virtually never diagnosed before birth. Jaundice is usually the only sign in mild and moderately severe HDN and it is rarely sufficiently severe to require exchange transfusion. Occasionally mild anaemia is present or may develop shortly after birth. The diagnosis is based on laboratory investigations.

Laboratory investigations
Serological studies on the mother demonstrate that she is blood group O and has a high titre of IgG anti-A or anti-B antibodies. The baby is blood group A or B. The direct antiglobulin test on the baby's red cells is sometimes positive; more often anti-A or anti-B may be eluted from the baby's red cells. Free anti-A or anti-B may be present in the baby's serum. Exceptionally, the mother has blood group A_2 and has a high titre of anti-A_1 while the baby is group A_1.

Haematological tests show mild to moderate anaemia. Microspherocytes and nucleated red cells are present in the peripheral blood film and the reticulocyte count is higher than normal.

Hyperbilirubinaemia develops more slowly and reaches the peak later than in HDN due to anti-D antibody. The insidious development of jaundice and the negative direct antiglobulin test should not preclude the diagnosis of HDN.

Management
The indication for exchange transfusion is rising serum bilirubin concentration which should not be allowed to exceed 250 μmol/l. For details of exchange transfusion see p. 34. There is no prevention for HDN due to ABO incompatibility.

HAEMOLYTIC DISEASE OF THE NEWBORN DUE TO ANTIBODIES AGAINST OTHER RED CELL ANTIGENS

Almost every antibody which occurs as IgG immunoglobulin and has a specificity against one of the red cell antigens, has been implicated in HDN. After anti-D, and anti-A and anti-B the most commonly found antibody causing HDN is anti-K. The pathogenesis, clinical presentation, laboratory investigations and management of HDN due to anti-K, and indeed all the other antibodies, are essentially the same as those for Rh(D) incompatibility. However, HDN is usually mild and only rarely will the affected baby require exchange transfusion. Exceptionally, severe forms of HDN may require antenatal management (maternal plasma exchanges, amniocentesis, intrauterine transfusions and early elective delivery) similar to that described for Rh HDN.

ALLOIMMUNE NEONATAL THROMBOCYTOPENIA

Definition
A transient severe thrombocytopenia in the newborn due to platelet destruction by maternal alloantibody.

Pathogenesis
The mother does not possess the platelet antigen which the baby has, usually Pl^{A1}, and she has been immunised by transfusion or pregnancy previously, and produces anti-Pl^{A1} alloantibody. The antibody crosses the placenta and destroys the baby's Pl^{A1}-positive platelets through complement mediated lysis or more often by coating platelets which are subsequently phagocytosed in the mononuclear phagocyte system. This is a rare condition; even more rare is neonatal thrombocytopenia caused by antibodies to other platelet antigens or HLA antigens.

Clinical presentation
In mildly affected infants a slightly reduced platelet count (50 to 100 × 10^9/l) may be the only sign. In the more severely affected baby generalised petechiae and mucosal bleeding are evident immediately after birth. Some 10% of severely affected infants suffer from CNS haemorrhage. Thrombocytopenia may persist for up to three months. The most critical period for the baby is at the time of birth and during the first week of life.

   Diagnosis is made after the birth of the first affected child. The baby has thrombocytopenia with normal numbers and maturation of megakaryocytes in the bone marrow. The mother has a normal platelet count, no history of ITP, and is almost invariably Pl^{A1} negative. The diagnosis is confirmed by demonstrating the presence of the antiplatelet antibody with Pl^{A1} specificity in the mother's serum. Differential diagnosis is presented in Table 13.5.

Management
Mildly affected infants without any sign of bleeding do not require treatment. The severely affected, at high risk of CNS haemorrhage, should be given platelets. There is little or no response to random donor platelets, since they will be Pl^{A1} positive. Three approaches to platelet transfusion can be used in order of preference:
   1. administration of Pl^{A1}-negative platelet concentrates;
   2. administration of platelet concentrate obtained by platelet apheresis from the mother. Platelets should be gently washed to remove the antibody and resuspended in AB Rh-negative plasma.
   3. If Pl^{A1}-negative platelets are not available and the mother cannot undergo platelet apheresis, the baby should have an

Table 13.5 Differential diagnosis of alloimmune neonatal thrombocytopenia

Condition	In the Baby			In the Mother	
	Bone marrow megakaryocytes	Coagulation screen		Typical finding	Platelet antibodies in the serum
Alloimmune neonatal thrombocytopenia	normal number	normal		Pl^{A1} negative	anti-Pl^{A1}
Autoimmune neonatal thrombocytopenia	normal number	normal		ITP	anti-platelet autoantibody
Congenital amegakaryocytic thrombocytopenia	absent*	normal		normal	none
Disseminated intravascular coagulation**	normal number+	abnormal		normal	none

* Other congenital abnormalities (usually of bones) are common.
** Associated with other disease or as a result of difficult birth
+ Bone marrow aspiration is usually not carried out.

exchange transfusion to remove the antiplatelet antibody and it should receive random donor platelet concentrates.

Pl^{A1}-negative platelets survive eight to nine days in the baby's circulation, when the platelet count becomes very low again. Nevertheless, repeated platelet transfusion is rarely needed after the first week of life, unless the baby has other medical problems. The duration of thrombocytopenia is variable, but does not exceed three months.

When a mother has had one affected baby, the chances of having another affected baby are very high. Tests on mother's blood cannot predict whether the baby will be affected. To protect a high risk unborn baby steroids are administered in high doses to the mother immediately before and during labour and care is taken to avoid trauma to the baby during delivery.

ALLOIMMUNE NEONATAL NEUTROPENIA

Definition
This is a disorder due to placental transfer of anti-NA1, –NA2, –NB1 or, rarely, –HLA antibodies. Mild neonatal neutropenia is not uncommon, but severe cases are quite rare.

Clinical presentation
In a severely affected infant profound neutropenia is evident at birth and persists for up to two weeks. Clinical manifestations include infections of the skin, umbilical stump, respiratory and urinary tracts, as well as septicaemia. The diagnosis is made on the basis of *serological studies* of the mother's white cells and serum. The serum contains strong leucoagglutinins of anti-NA1, –NA2 or more rarely, –NB1 specificity. Other congenital neutropenias must be considered in differential diagnosis (Table 13.6).

Table 13.6 Differential diagnosis of alloimmune neonatal neutropenia

Condition	Bone marrow	Typical features Lymphoid cells in the blood	Duration of neutropenia
Alloimmune neonatal neutropenia	normal appearance	normal numbers	up to 2 weeks
Kostman's syndrome	absent myeloid precursors	low numbers or absent	life-long
Reticular dysgenesis	absent myeloid precursors	normal (monocytosis and eosinophilia)	life-long
Severe infections	absent more mature myeloid cells	transient lymphocytopenia may occur	normalisation of the neutrophil count as soon as infection subsides

Management

Granulocyte transfusion is only exceptionally required, as neutropenia is transient and infections are usually controlled by appropriate antibiotics. If granulocyte transfusion is considered to be essential, for example in severe septicaemia, maternal leucocytes should be harvested and given to the baby.

REFERENCES

American Association of Blood Banks, Washington 1981 Technical manual of the American Association of Blood Banks, 8th end.
Baehner R L, Boxer L A 1981 Disorders of granulopoiesis and granulocyte function. In: Nathan D G, Oski F A (eds) Hematology of infancy and childhood, 2nd edn. Saunders, Philadelphia, ch 25, p 838–865
Buchanan G R 1981 Haemorrhagic diseases. In: Nathan D G, Oski F A (eds) Hematology of infancy and childhood, 2nd edn. W B Saunders Company, Philadelphia, ch 5, p 119–143
Department of Health and Social Security 1984 Notes on transfusion
Department of Health and Social Security 1976 SMAC Memorandum on haemolytic diseases of the newborn
Department of Health and Social Security 1981 SMAC Memorandum on haemolytic disease of the newborn. Addendum
Gartner L M 1981 Disorders of bilirubin metabolism. In: Nathan D G, Oski F A (eds) Hematology of infancy and childhood, 2nd edn. Saunders, Philadelphia, ch 4, p 86–118
Mollison P L 1983 Blood transfusion in clinical medicine, 7th edn. Blackwell Scientific, Oxford
Plapp F V, Beck M L 1984 Transfusion support in the management of immune haemolytic disorders. In: Bayer W L (ed) Blood transfusion and blood banking. Clinics in Haematology 13: 167–183
Proceedings of the McMaster Conference on Prevention of Rh Immunization 1979 Vox Sanguinis 36: 50–64
Tovey L A D 1982 Rh prophylaxis in England and Wales: the present position. In: Frigoletto F D Jr, Jewett J F, Konugres A A (eds) Rh hemolytic disease. New strategy for eradication. Hall Medical, Boston
Zipursky A 1981 Isoimmune hemolytic diseases. In: Nathan D G, Oski F A (eds) Hematology of infancy and childhood, 2nd edn. Saunders, Philadelphia, ch 3, p 50–85

14. ACQUIRED IMMUNO-HAEMATOLOGICAL DISEASES: LABORATORY INVESTIGATION AND BLOOD TRANSFUSION

Each of the three haemopoietic cell lines may be the target of an immune process with subsequent shortened cell survival. This chapter deals with the diagnostic procedures and problems associated with transfusion of blood or blood components in patients with such antibody mediated diseases.

IMMUNE HAEMOLYTIC ANAEMIA

Immune haemolytic anaemia can be caused by an autoantibody produced by the patient and reacting against an antigenic determinant(s) on his own red cells, by a drug induced antibody, or it can be a manifestation of the red cell abnormality such as in paroxysmal nocturnal haemoglobinuria.

Autoimmune haemolytic anaemia (AIHA)

Two distinct clinical entities of AIHA exist, one with cold reacting antibodies and the other with warm reacting antibodies.

AIHA with cold reacting antibodies

Definition and pathological physiology
In AIHA with cold reacting antibody, the antibody, usually IgM, reacts with red cells best at temperatures below 37°C. The reaction permits the fixation of complement to the red cell membrane and subsequent intravascular destruction of the red cell by complement. Manifestations of the disease are on the one hand caused by haemolysis: haemoglobinaemia, haemoglobinuria and anaemia, and on the other hand by agglutination of red cells: acrocyanosis, vasculitic lesions and even gangrene. These manifestations are more marked in cold ambient temperatures.

Clinical syndromes
    1. Cold haemagglutinin disease may be idiopathic (chronic cold haemagglutinin disease, CHAD) or secondary to lymphoproliferative conditions (chronic lymphocytic leukaemia, lymphoma) and infections, particularly in children, caused by *Mycoplasma pneumoniae*, cytomegalovirus, infectious mononucleosis, etc.
    2. Paroxysmal cold haemoglobinuria is caused by an antibody

(Donath-Landsteiner) which reacts reacts in the cold and promotes the fixation of complement. Complement mediated lysis occurs at body temperature. It is usually associated with syphilis in adults and viral infections in children.

The diagnosis is established by demonstrating the presence of haemolysis, the presence of a cold reacting antibody in the plasma and the determination of its properties. *Harmless* cold reacting antibodies are present in a low titre, react at temperatures less than 25°C and do not cause haemolysis. *Harmful* cold reacting antibodies are present in a high titre, have a thermal amplitude of reaction which approaches 37°C or are capable of reacting at 37°C, and cause haemolysis. Some properties of cold reacting antibodies are listed in Table 14.1.

Blood transfusion problems encountered in AIHA with cold reacting antibodies are related to the blood grouping and compatibility testing and to the choice of blood and transfusion procedure.

1. *Blood grouping and compatibility* testing can be extremely difficult and should be carried out strictly at 37°C (for details see a manual of laboratory procedures). In the *choice of blood* for transfusion one should select a product with the least volume of plasma as a source of complement: frozen and thawed or washed red cells, and when these are not available, concentrated red cells should be prepared from blood nearing its expiry date.

2. *Transfusion procedure* Warm blood, preferably using an in-line blood warmer, and transfuse slowly. Keep the patient warm, observe half-hourly, keep a fluid balance chart and check the urine regularly for haemoglobinuria. Should haemoglobin appear in the urine, slow down the transfusion or stop it. Patients with a history of febrile and allergic reactions should receive antihistamines and hydrocortisone prior to transfusion (p. 97). Note that these drugs have no effect on haemolysis.

Transfusion to patients with harmless cold reacting antibodies is unlikely to provoke a haemolytic transfusion reaction. Nevertheless, it is advisable to use warmed blood when transfusing such patients. Potential problems associated with cardiopulmonary bypass in such patients are discussed on p. 39.

AIHA with warm reacting antibodies

Definition and pathological physiology
The warm reacting antibodies in AIHA are IgG immunoglobulins reacting best at 37°C. The antibody coats the red cells causing their sequestration in the spleen and liver, where they are phagocytosed by the macrophages. This results in anaemia, spherocytosis, raised reticulocyte count and splenomegaly.

Clinical syndromes
Most cases are idiopathic and run a chronic course. Occasionally fulminant and life-threatening haemolysis is the first presentation of the

Table 14.1 Some properties of cold reacting autoantibodies

Antibody and clinical syndrome	Ig class	Specificity	In vitro effect	In vivo effect
Normal incomplete antibody	not an immunoglobulin	anti-H	enables complement fixation by normal red cells	harmless
Normal cold autoantibody	IgM (low titre)	anti-I	coats and agglutinates red cells	harmless
Autoantibody found in CHAD	IgM	anti-I, rarely anti-Pr*	agglutinates red cells at low temperature, causes complement mediated haemolysis at 37°C	haemolytic anaemia, Raynaud's phenomen, vasculitic lesions and gangrene
Autoantibody in *M.pneumoniae*	IgM	anti-I	agglutinates red cells, occasionally haemolytic	occasionally haemolytic anaemia
Autoantibody in infectious mononucleosis	IgM	anti-i	agglutinates red cells, occasionally haemolytic	occasionally haemolytic anaemia
Autoantibody in CLL and lymphoma	IgM	anti-i	agglutinates red cells, occasionally haemolytic	occasionally haemolytic anaemia
Donath-Landsteiner autoantibody in paroxysmal cold haemoglobinuria	IgG	anti-P	agglutinates red cells, occasionally haemolytic	haemolytic anaemia

* A group of antigens present on *all* red cells, which are easily destroyed by enzyme treatement

disease. A proportion of cases is associated with lymphoproliferative and collagen diseases. In children, transient haemolytic anaemia may occur after a viral infection. Some tumours, in particular ovarian, are associated with warm reacting antibodies.

Diagnosis is established on the basis of a positive direct antiglobulin test (DAT) in the presence of haemolytic anaemia. Using specific antiglobulin reagents, molecules of IgG alone or IgG and components of complement can be demonstrated on the red cells. In the majority of cases the warm reacting antibody has no specificity. In the remainder of cases the antibody has specificity of an antigen in the Rh system, usually anti-e, or another specificity such as anti-Wr^a.

Note that a positive DAT does not mean autoimmune haemolysis unless evidence of shortened red cell survival is present. A small number of healthy people have positive DATs without any evidence of haemolysis.

Blood transfusion

1. *Blood grouping and compatibility testing* may be extremely difficult. In addition a strong warm reacting antibody may mask the presence of alloantibodies such as anti-K, anti-Jk^a or others (for details of testing consult a manual on laboratory procedures).

   Choice of blood. If the autoantibody has a specificity, the red cells lacking the corresponding antigen should be selected for transfusion. For example, a patient with warm reacting anti-e antibody should be transfused with compatible group ABO red cells of R_2R_2 (cDE/cDE) phenotype. In most instances, however, the antibody has no specificity and reacts equally strongly with the patient's own red cells and donors' red cells. Such blood is called 'least incompatible' blood. It is also helpful to give blood with the least possible concentration of complement. Therefore frozen and thawed or washed red cells should be used. If these are not available, concentrated red cells should be prepared from units of blood nearing expiry date.

2. *Transfusion procedure* Although transfusion in fulminant haemolytic anaemia is a very dangerous procedure which may precipitate renal or cardiac failure, or disseminated intravascular coagulation, it should not be withheld from a severely anaemic patient, for whom it may be life saving.

   Transfuse not more than one unit of 'least incompatible' blood over a period of four to eight hours. Observe the patient closely at 15 min intervals and keep a fluid balance chart. Test the urine for haemoglobinuria and check the blood count and coagulation status. Slow the transfusion or stop if there is increasing dyspnoea, hypotension, fever or clinical or laboratory evidence of disseminated intravascular coagulation. If no untoward reaction has occurred continue transfusing one unit of blood daily until a haemoglobin concentration of 7 to 8 g/dl is reached. If the patient is not already on high dose steroids give hydrocortisone 100 to 200 mg i.v. prior to each unit of blood.

Other procedures which may be beneficial are plasma exchange, emergency splenectomy and administration of immunosuppressive drugs.

Blood transfusion in patients with chronic immune haemolytic anaemia
It is occasionally necessary to transfuse such patients to prevent cardiac failure or prior to an operation. The likelihood of serious untoward reactions to transfusion is less than in patients with fulminant haemolysis but all the precautions described above should be taken.

Blood transfusion in patients with positive DAT and without evidence of haemolysis
Patients with positive DAT but without evidence of haemolysis, who require blood transfusion for non-haematological reasons, are unlikely to have severe untoward transfusion reactions. However, on compatibility testing only 'least incompatible' blood may be available and the following precautions should be taken:

Administer intravenously an antihistamine preparation (e.g. chlorpheniramine, Piriton, 10 mg) and hydrocortisone (100 mg), prior to transfusion; transfuse slowly using an in-line blood warmer.

Observe the patient closely at 30 min intervals and check the temperature and blood pressure.

Keep a fluid balance chart, test the urine for haemoglobin and bilirubin at least once during and at the end of the transfusion.

Check the haemoglobin concentration at the end of the transfusion to confirm that the expected rise has been achieved.

Drug induced immune haemolytic anaemia

Definition and pathological physiology
In this condition a drug induced immune haemolysis is responsible for the destruction of red cells. Three mechanisms of red cell destruction are recognised:

1. An immune complex of the drug and the antibody to it activate complement on the surface of red cells causing lysis. This type of haemolysis is brisk but usually short lived. Drugs commonly implicated are quinine, quinidine, PAS, sulphonamides and rifampicin.

2. The drug is adsorbed onto the red cell membrane; antibodies to the drug interact with it causing lysis of the 'innocent bystander' — the red cell. Haemolytic anaemia of moderate severity usually ensues. Drugs commonly involved are penicillins and cephalosporins given in high dose.

3. The drug induces production of autoantibodies against red

cell antigens, and true autoimmune haemolytic anaemia, of variable severity, occurs. α-methyldopa is an example of such a drug.

Diagnosis is based on the history of drug administration, a positive DAT and the presence of haemolytic anaemia. For details of serological investigations see a manual of laboratory procedures. Haemolysis ceases as soon as the drug is discontinued, except in α-methyldopa induced haemolytic anaemia where haemolysis persists for three months or longer after discontinuing the drug.

Blood transfusion
Blood grouping and compatibility testing usually do not present a problem. Note that the donor's red cells, once in the circulation, will be affected by the haemolytic mechanism in the same way as the recipient's red cells. For transfusion to a patient with α-methyldopa induced haemolytic anaemia use 'least incompatible' blood and follow the procedure described on p. 141. Reactions to blood are rare and usually mild.

PAROXYSMAL NOCTURNAL HAEMOGLOBINURIA

Definition and pathological physiology
Paroxysmal nocturnal haemoglobinuria (PNH) is a disorder of haemopoietic stem cells. All cells produced by an abnormal clone(s) have a membrane defect which renders them susceptible to lysis by complement. The cardinal feature of PNH is haemolytic anaemia due to intravascular lysis of red cells.

Diagnosis is made by demonstrating that the patient's red cells are unusually susceptible to lysis by complement. The test used is Ham's test in which complement is activated by acidified serum; other means of activating complement are the use of reduced ionic strength medium in which to incubate the red cells, insulin, snake venom, etc.

Blood transfusion
Patients with PNH almost invariably react to transfusion of blood: rigors, abdominal pain, diarrhoea, vomiting, haemoglobinuria and failure to achieve the expected rise of haemoglobin concentration are common. When blood transfusion is required use frozen and thawed or washed red cells. It is advisable to administer an antihistamine and hydrocortisone prior to transfusion and to follow the procedure described on p. 141.

IMMUNE THROMBOCYTOPENIAS

Idiopathic thrombocytopenic purpura (ITP)

Definition and pathological physiology
ITP is a disease brought about by an autoantibody directed against platelets. The autoantibody is an IgG immunoglobulin which coats

platelets to cause sequestration in the reticulo-endothelial system with subsequent phagocytosis by the macrophages.

Clinical syndromes

Two well differentiated forms of ITP exist: acute post viral thrombocytopenia of childhood, and the chronic ITP of adults. The first condition runs a self limiting course of a few weeks or months, whereas the second runs a chronic course over many years. A proportion of adult cases are associated with SLE, other collagen disorders and with lymphoproliferative diseases.

Diagnositic procedures in the blood bank

In ITP platelets are coated with IgG, and in some cases free antiplatelet antibody can be found in serum. The following tests are used to demonstrate the platelet antibody: antiglobulin consumption test, platelet immunofluorescence test, radioactive antiglobulin consumption test, and immunoperoxidase assay. All these tests are technically complex and occasionally show false positive results; for example, platelet coating with IgG can be demonstrated in rheumatoid arthritis, chronic lymphatic leukaemia, etc, in the absence of thrombocytopenia. Note that the diagnosis of ITP is made on the basis of haematological (low platelet count, normal megakaryocytes in the bone marrow), biochemical (absence of abnormalities), and clinical observations, and that serological tests are of contributory value only.

Platelet transfusion in ITP is only used in dire emergency. Since the platelet antibody is directed against all platelets, the routine use of platelet transfusion is not indicated, as the platelets will be rapidly destroyed. However, in a life-threatening episode, such as CNS haemorrhage, massive gastrointestinal bleed or emergency splenectomy, platelet transfusion should be given (p. 56).

ITP in pregnancy

The IgG antiplatelet antibody may cross the placenta and cause severe thrombocytopenia in the baby. Neonatal thrombocytopenia is common when the mother's platelet count is low; even when the mother is in remission and with a normal platelet count, some 10–15% of such babies are born with thrombocytopenia. In the mildly affected infants the only abnormality is a slightly reduced platelet count (around $50 \times 10^9/l$). Severely affected babies have widespread purpura, petechiae, bruising and may bleed into the gastrointestinal tract or CNS. Thrombocytopenia persists for up to three months, but the major risk is during the first week of life. The management of an asymptomatic baby with low platelet count only does not require active measures. If the baby is severely affected, management consists of exchange transfusion (to remove the maternal antibody) followed by platelet transfusion. It is not possible to predict from serological studies of the mother which infants will be severely affected. It is therefore wise to avoid birth trauma as much as possible. Administration of steroids to the mother immediately before and during delivery may have a protective effect against severe haemorrhage in the baby (see also p. 136).

Drug-induced immune thrombocytopenia

Definition and pathological physiology

Thrombocytopenia is caused by an immune process occurring only in the presence of a drug. Two mechanisms are responsible for the destruction of platelets:

1. The combination of the drug and a plasma protein stimulates antibody production. The antigen-antibody complex is bound to the platelet surface and the platelet is destroyed. This is the 'innocent bystander' mechanism.

2. The drug binds to an antigen on the platelet surface. The antibodies are produced against such a complex and carry both drug and platelet specificity.

A list of *drugs* commonly implicated in drug-induced immune thrombocytopenia is shown in Table 14.2.

Table 14.2 Drugs commonly implicated in immune thrombocytopenia

Quinidine
Quinine
Gold
Phenytoin
Sodium valproate
Sulphonamides
Penicillins
PAS
Rifampicine
Heparin
Aspirin

Diagnosis

The tests to detect drug dependent antiplatelet antibodies are of two kinds: simple tests which are relatively insensitive but when positive conclusively prove the diagnosis; and complex tests designed to detect minor alterations of the platelets; these tests are technically difficult, and their interpretation is not easy. In experienced hands they can be a useful diagnostic tool. A list of tests is given in Table 14.3.

Management

Platelet transfusion is not indicated unless there is a life threatening episode, as the donor's platelets will be destroyed rapidly in the patient's circulation.

Table 14.3 Tests used to detect drug dependent platelet antibodies

First line tests	*Second line tests*
Platelet agglutination	Complement fixation test
Platelet lysis	Antiglobulin consumption test
Clot retraction inhibition	PF3 availability
	Serotonin release measurement
	Inhibition of platelet aggregation

Post-transfusion purpura

Definition
Severe thrombocytopenia developing approximately one week after blood transfusion, due to platelet destruction by alloantibodies.

Pathological physiology
Most cases have occurred in Pl^{A1}-negative women who develop anti-Pl^{A1}, but other platelet specific antigens may also be involved. The mechanism by which anti-Pl^{A1} destroys Pl^{A1}-negative platelets of the affected individual is not known. Two explanations have been suggested: one that the antibody cross-reacts with other Pl^{A1}-related determinants to cause lysis of Pl^{A1}-negative platelets, and the other that the transfusion of Pl^{A1}-positive blood that precedes the onset of purpura induces the synthesis of Pl^{A1} substance and its uptake by platelets. Such transiently 'positive' platlets are then destroyed by the antibody.

The clinical picture is that of a severe bleeding disorder with a sudden onset one week after blood transfusion. Thrombocytopenia persists for a period of ten days to two months.

The diagnosis is suspected on the basis of time elapsed after transfusion and confirmed by finding strong anti-platelet antibodies, usually anti-Pl^{A1} in the patient who is almost invariably Pl^{A1} negative.

Management
Treatment with steroids is ineffective. Platelet transfusion, even with Pl^{A1}-negative platelets is also of no avail, since the transfused platelets are rapidly destroyed. Some reports indicate that removal of antibody by plasmapheresis appears to ameliorate the bleeding and to shorten the duration of thrombocytopenia. In a life threatening situation give Pl^{A1}-negative platelets (if available) to prevent further sensitisation. Recently high dose intravenous immunoglobulin (p. 75) has been used with success.

IMMUNE NEUTROPENIA

Autoimmune neutropenia

Definition
Neutropenia due to the destruction of neutrophil granulocytes by an autoantibody.

Clinical picture
This is an uncommon syndrome, sometimes associated with other autoimmune diseases and Felty's syndrome. There is a variable degree of neutropenia and the patient has a relatively mild disease which includes malaise, mouth ulcers, pharyngitis or cellulitis.

Diagnosis
Normal myeloid precursors are increased in the bone marrow. The serum

shows an anti-neutrophil antibody usually without specificity, but some cases of anti-NA2 antibodies have been described.

Management is conservative.

Autoimmune neutropenia and pregnancy
Women with autoimmune neutropenia may give birth to children with severe neonatal neutropenia associated with infections. For their management see p. 137.

Drug induced immune neutropenia

Definition and pathological physiology
Neutropenia due to a drug-induced immune destruction of neutrophil granulocytes. The immune reaction involving neutrophils is usually of very acute onset and associated with rapid lysis of target cells — neutrophils. The list of drugs commonly implicated is given in Table 14.4.

Table 14.4 Drugs associated with immune neutropenia*

Analgesics:	Aminopyrine**
	Phenylbutazone
Antibiotics:	Tetracycline
	Chloramphenicol
	Methicillin
Antihistamines:	Chlorpheniramine
	Promethazine
Antithyroid drugs:	Propylthiouracil
	Carbimazole
Antidiabetic drugs:	Tolbutamide
Tranquilisers:	Prochlorperazine
	Promazine
	Chlorpromazine
	Meprobamate
Other drugs:	Barbiturates
	Penicillamine
	Cimetidine
	Phenindione

* The list is not complete and in some instances a combination of immune mechanism and marrow suppression may be responsible for neutropenia.
** Not available in the U.K.

Clinical picture
There is a sudden onset of violent chills, fever, and sometimes shock. Less often there is a severe focal infection such as pneumonia or pharyngitis. A proportion of patients recover on withdrawal of the drug.

Diagnosis may be difficult since it is not always possible to demonstrate leukoagglutinins. Re-challenge with the suspected drug should not be undertaken unless the drug is essential for the patient's future management, because it may cause severe, even fatal, reactions.

Management
Treatment of infection is with antibiotics. Granulocyte transfusions are contraindicated since they may cause serious anaphylactic reaction or lung

infiltrates (see p. 61). In cases of overwhelming sepsis with the diagnosis in doubt, granulocyte transfusion may be considered as a 'last ditch' measure.

REFERENCES

British National Formulary 1984 British Medical Association and the Pharmaceutical Society of Great Britain, London, Number 8
Hoffbrand A V, Lewis S M (eds) 1981 Postgraduate haematology, 2nd edn. Heinemann, London
Huestis D W, Bove J R, Busch S 1981 Practical blood transfusion. Little, Brown, Boston
Ingram G I C, Brozović M, Slater N G P 1982 Bleeding disorders. Investigation and management, 2nd edn. Blackwell Scientific, Oxford
Minchinton R M, Waters A H 1984 The occurrence and significance of neutrophil antibodies. British Journal of Haematology 56: 521–528
Petz L D, Swisher S (eds) 1981 Clinical practice of blood transfusion. Churchill Livingstone, Edinburgh
Woods V L Jr, McMillan R 1984 Platelet antigens in chronic ITP. British Journal of Haematology 57: 1–4

15. APHERESIS

Apheresis (or haemapheresis) is the collection of blood from a donor or patient, separation and removal of a cellular component(s) and/or plasma and the return of the remaining blood constituents. Apheresis is used for *harvesting* cell components and plasma from healthy donors and in the *treatment* of patients by the removal of abnormal or harmful blood constituents from the circulation.

Cytapheresis is a procedure by which the cellular elements of the blood, platelets (platelet apheresis, thrombocytapheresis), leucocytes (leucapheresis), lymphocytes (lymphocytapheresis) or red cells (erythrocytapheresis), are selectively removed from the blood.

Plasmapheresis is the selective removal of plasma. It is performed either to collect plasma (up to 600 ml) from a healthy donor, without fluid replacement, or as plasma exchange in a patient, when several litres of plasma are removed and replaced by crystalloid and protein solutions. Plasmapheresis is by far the most frequently used procedure, followed by plateletapheresis and to a lesser extent by leucapheresis.

PROCEDURES

Manual apheresis

Manual apheresis from a donor is carried out by collecting 450 ml of blood into a multiple pack with anticoagulant; the pack is centrifuged, plasma (or platelet rich plasma or buffy coat) is transferred to a satellite pack, and the concentrated red cells are resuspended in saline and rapidly returned to the donor through the collection needle, kept open by a saline drip. The procedure yields about 250 ml of plasma (and one unit of platelet concentrate or buffy coat). It can be repeated once (double manual apheresis).

Untoward effects of manual apheresis, in addition to those associated with blood donation are:

1. Bruising at the needle site is more frequent than in blood donation.
2. Failure to return the red cells, either because they are lost during processing or because the venous access becomes

blocked. In that case the donor should not resume plasmapheresis until four to eight weeks have elapsed.

3. Return of wrongly identified red cells. This is the most serious hazard of manual apheresis, which may give rise to alloimmunisation of the donor as well as serious haemolytic transfusion reaction. A protocol for identification of the donor's red cells prior to return must be established and strictly adhered to in every apheresis clinic.

Comment
Manual apheresis is a simple and inexpensive procedure primarily used for harvesting plasma for fractionation, but should be considered both for harvesting of cells and as a therapeutic procedure, where blood cell processors are not available.

Table 15.1 Blood cell processors used for apheresis

Blood cell processors employing centrifugation
Continuous flow centrifugation (CFC):
Aminco Celltrifuge
Cobe 2997 Blood Cell Processor
Fenwal Celltrifuge II
Fenwal CS-3000 Blood Cell Processor
Intermittent flow centrifugation (IFC):
Haemonetics-30
Haemonetics-50*
Haemonetics-V50
Haemonetics PCS*
Dideco Progress 90
Blood cell processors employing plasmafiltration
Cobe Centry TPE system
Organon Teknika with Curesis filter
Organon Teknika with Plasmapur filter*
Hemoscience Autopheresis-C**
Fenwal PS-400 with CPS-10 filter
Dideco BT 798 Viva

 * Used for plasma-harvesting only
** Undergoing trials for plasma-harvesting

Apheresis using blood cell processors

When apheresis using a blood cell processor (cell separator) is carried out the donor (or the patient) remains attached to the processor throughout the procedure. Available processors are listed in Table 15.1; anticoagulant and disposable kit with replacement fluids are also required, the latter when more than 600 ml of plasma and cell suspension are to be collected.

Blood cell processors

Centrifugal blood cell processors
Separation of cells and plasma is achieved by centrifugation of blood in a separation chamber. There are several types of separation chambers: a spinning bowl (Haemonetics system), rotary belt (Cobe 2997 Blood Cell Processor, previously marketed as IBM 2997 Blood Cell Processor), or a

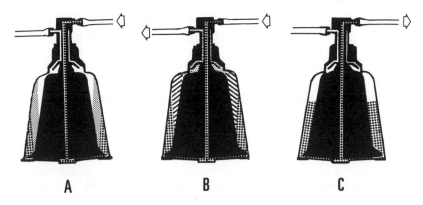

Fig. 15.1 Separating chamber and seal of the Haemonetics-30 Cell Separator.
(A) Anticoagulated blood is pumped into the rotary bowl and plasma separation begins.
(B) As the bowl fills component layers are formed. Platelet poor plasma (finely stippled),
platelet rich plasma and leucocyte (hatched) are sequentially expelled. (C) When the bowl is
full of red cells (stippled) centrifugation stops, and red cells are pumped into a bag for
reinfusion by gravity. (Redrawn from: Apheresis Systems, Haemonetics Corporation, with kind
permission of Haemonetics (UK) Limited)

system of two separation packs (Travenol CS-3000 Blood Processor).
Each type of separation chamber has its own specially designed connector
to provide continuity between the rotary and stationary parts (Fig. 15.1,
15.2 and 15.3).

When blood is withdrawn from and returned to the donor in a
continuous flow the procedure is conventionally called continuous flow
centrifugation (CFC), and when there is an intermittent flow the
procedure is called intermittent flow centrifugation (IFC). Plasmafiltration
too can be carried out as a continuous or intermittent procedure. CFC
processors require venous access at two sites, while IFC processors can
operate with venous access at either one or two sites.

Filtration leucapheresis employs the property of nylon fibre filters
(Leuko-Pak, Travenol) to retain granulocytes from heparinised blood in
the presence of calcium ions. The granulocytes are then harvested from
the filter by elution. It is not in use in Britain.

Plasma filtration separators use filters of either hollow fibre or flat
membranes. The membrane has numerous holes of about 0.6 μ in
diameter. The blood flows on one side of the membrane and when
sufficient transmembrane pressure is achieved plasma seeps through the
holes.

Safety features of blood cell processors
All blood cell processors must have the following safety features:
1. A blood flow monitor to prevent the pump from drawing
   blood from the donor at a rate exceeding that of the donor's
   venous flow.
2. A return flow pressure monitor to stop the return of blood
   when the flow is obstructed or the vein occluded. The

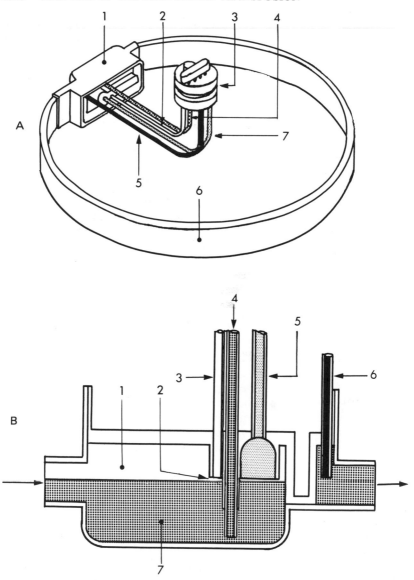

Fig. 15.2 Single stage collection belt and chamber (Cobe Model 302) of the Cobe 2997 Blood Cell Processor. (A) Anticoagulated blood enters the rotary belt through whole blood input tube (5), travels through the separation channel (6) and reaches the separation chamber (1) from where the components are harvested. White cell tube (2); seal assembly which provides the continuity between the rotary and the stationary parts (3); packed red cell tube (4); interface positioning port (plasma tube) (7). (B) Cross-section of the collection chamber. Arrows indicate the flow of blood. Plasma (1); buffy coat (2); white cell collection port (3); packed red cell port (4); interface positioning port (plasma tube) (5); whole blood input tube (6); packed red cells (7). (Redrawn from: Cobe 2997 Blood Cell Processor, Technical Information, with kind permission of Cobe Laboratories, Inc.)

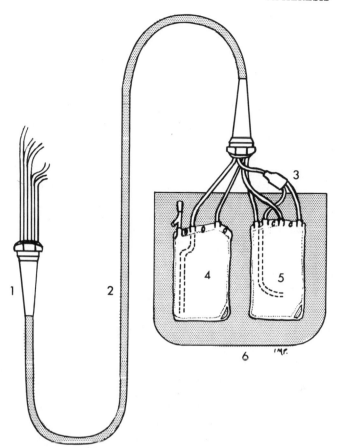

Fig. 15.3 Separation container, collection container and multiple lumen tubing of the Fenwal CS-3000 Blood Cell Separator. The stationary part (pumps, bubble trap detector, saline and anticoagulant containers, and associated tubing) are not shown in this figure with the exception of the upper hexagonal strain relief position (1). This specially designed, seal-less connection links the multiple lumen tubing (2) to the lower hexagonal strain position (3). The design of the cell separator enables the tube to twist and untwist during centrifugation. Whole blood enters the separation container (5) through one of the lumens in the multiple lumen tubing; platelet rich plasma with or without leucocytes is separated by centrifugation and returned into the collection container (4) via the stationary part not shown. The separation and collection containers are centrifuged within the centrifuge chamber (6). (Redrawn from: Apheresis kit, Fenwal Laboratories, 8-19-3-592AA, 1979, with kind permission of Travenol Laboratories Limited)

monitor is not required in systems which return blood by gravity.

3. A bubble detector to detect air in the return line, to stop the return pump and sound the alarm. The bubble detector is not required in systems which return blood by gravity.

4. All blood processors must be programmed to enter the stand-by mode when power is resumed following a power failure.
5. It is desirable but not essential that blood in the extracorporeal circuit can be returned manually to the donor if the power fails or if the machine breaks down.

Apheresis kits

Apheresis kits consist of the separation chamber and all connecting lines. They are disposable, made for 'once only' use. Appropriate kits are supplied by each of the manufacturers of blood cell processors.

Anticoagulant solutions

1. Anticoagulants containing citrate, either ACD(A) or ACD(B), are used for all apheresis procedures with the exception of filtration leucapheresis, with a ratio of anticoagulant to blood between 1:8 and 1:12. Other formulations may be used for special and research purposes or when the anticoagulant to blood ratio is in the range from 1:15 to 1:25.
2. Heparin may be used for therapeutic apheresis of patients, administered intravenously to the patient as an initial dose or by continuous infusion during the procedure. The dose must be sufficient to prevent coagulation of blood in the extracorporeal circuit, and will depend on the protocol and the duration of apheresis. Usually it is between 10 000 and 20 000 i.u. Heparin is not recommended for use in healthy donors, with the exception of those undergoing filtration leucapheresis, because of the possibility of rare but potentially serious complications. There may be immediate untoward reactions, hypersensitivity reactions, anaphylactic shock and mild haemolysis; heparin induced thrombocytopenia may present later.

Extracorporeal volume of blood

In CFC blood cell processors the extracorporeal volume does not exceed 200 ml and the withdrawal and return of blood are perfectly matched throughout the procedure. Thus the person undergoing apheresis is not subjected to changes in circulatory volume. In IFC blood cell processors the extracorporeal volume may exceed 500 ml, but a skilful operator can protect the patient from gross changes of the circulatory volume by balancing carefully the rates of blood withdrawal and return of red cells and replacement solutions.

Hazards of apheresis

Harvesting procedures carried out on healthy donors are in general safe. Untoward reactions are due to citrate toxicity and are usually mild and transient (see below). Leucapheresis is more frequently associated with untoward reactions, although the incidence is still less than 1%. These reactions are due to steroid premedication and use of sedimenting agents.

Hazards of therapeutic apheresis are related to citrate toxicity, changes in the circulation volume, problems with venous access, loss of platelets and/or plasma proteins and the use of replacement fluids.

1. Citrate toxicity has been observed in all types of apheresis procedures with frequency of up to 10%; this is not surprising since the volume of blood processed is usually between 2 and 6 l. A very serious technical error will be made if the pack with anticoagulant instead of the saline pack is connected to the return line; this will lead to severe citrate toxicity immediately after starting the procedure. For details of citrate toxicity see p. 103.

2. Changes in the circulatory volume may precipitate severe hypotensive episodes or cardiac failure.

3. Establishing venous access may be difficult and on occasions cannulation of the superior vena cava, catheterisation of the femoral vein or formation of an arterio-venous shunt may be required.

4. Fluid replacement, in particular with fresh frozen plasma, may cause citrate toxicity, as well as allergic or anaphylactoid reactions (see p. 98). Fresh frozen plasma also carries the risk of transmitting hepatitis.

5. The loss of platelets, coagulation factors and plasma proteins is regularly seen in therapeutic procedures. However, it is rarely associated with impaired haemostasis as the recovery of the platelet count and coagulation factors is rapid, within one to two days. No corrective measures are required unless intensive and frequent plasma exchanges are carried out. FFP used as part of the replacement fluid will correct the deficiency of clotting factors and PPF that of albumin. Infection due to the loss of immunoglobulins has been reported only in exceptional situations.

Management of untoward effects

1. Effects of citrate toxicity are reduced by decreasing the rate of return of blood and replacement fluids which contain citrate, by giving saline more rapidly, and by providing calcium gluconate tablets. Administration of calcium gluconate intravenously is best avoided. Although cardiac arrhythmias are transient, facilities for resuscitation must be available in the apheresis clinic.

2. Keeping a fluid balance chart during apheresis will prevent serious reduction of the circulatory volume or fluid overload. Hypotension may quickly improve on increased rate of fluid return. Fluid overload responds to diuretics (see p. 102).

3. For the management of urticarial or anaphylactoid reactions to fresh frozen plasma see p. 99, 100.

APHERESIS OF DONORS

Guidelines and selection of donors

Guidelines for the use of blood cell separators in apheresis units in the UK are presented in *A Code of Practice for the Clinical Use of Blood Cell Separators* (DHSS, 1977). The Code makes recommendations regarding the selection, medical examination and care of donors, and the procedure for obtaining informed consent. The Code also contains information about the use and care of equipment, the frequency of use necessary to maintain a high standard of proficiency, associated hazards, the numbers, grades and training of staff and the physical and special resuscitation facilities which must be available if it is decided to install and operate a blood cell separator. Many other countries have prepared similar guidelines.

Selection of donors

In the transfusion centres apheresis donors are recruited from the ranks of regular blood donors. In hospital, apheresis donors are usually selected from the members of the patient's family and close friends. Some hospitals have their own apheresis panels.

Plasmapheresis

Plasma is collected by single or double manual plasmapheresis or by blood cell processors (Haemonetics 50 and V50 processors) or by plasmafiltration. Plasma collected by plasmapheresis is used as fresh frozen plasma for administration to patients or for fractionation and production of factor VIII concentrate, albumin or immunoglobulins. Recommendations in the UK limit the volume of plasma collected to 600 ml at any one time, not more frequently than once a fortnight and to a total volume not exceeding 15 l a year.

Platelet apheresis

Platelets are harvested by manual apheresis or by platelet apheresis using blood processors from random or selected donors. Selection of donors, methods of collection and properties of platelet concentrates are described in Chapter 5.

The yield of platelets collected is proportional to the donor's initial platelet count, the volume of blood processed and the protocol used.

Hazards for the donor

In addition to untoward reactions seen in other apheresis procedures, the platelet count is invariably reduced by platelet apheresis, but spontaneously returns to normal within the following few days. It is recommended that the count should not be reduced below 100×10^9/l and that platelets should not be donated more often than 12 times a year.

Donor panels
Whenever possible regular platelet apheresis donors should be tested for CMV antibodies, P1^{A1} antigen and HLA antigens.

Collection of granulocytes

Collection of granulocytes is carried out using blood cell processors, filtration leucapheresis and gravity leucapheresis. Methods of collection and properties of granulocyte concentrates are described in Chapter 6.

The yield of granulocytes collected depends on the initial granulocyte count and the volume of blood processed. The yield is improved by using a sedimenting agent, dextran or hydroxyethyl starch (HES), during centrifugation of blood, and by administering corticosteroids prior to leucapheresis for augmenting the granulocyte count.

Hazards for the donor
In addition to the untoward effects seen in other apheresis procedures, side effects associated with the infusion of dextran may be present: abdominal cramps, expansion of plasma volume, and retention of dextran by the mononuclear phagocyte system. A rare occurrence of lichen planus following repeated leucapheresis has been described.

Collection of young red cells

At present the collection of young red cells using a blood cell processor is a research procedure, since the evidence that the transfusion of young red cells extends the interval between transfusions in multitransfused patients has not been substantiated.

THERAPEUTIC APHERESIS

Plasma exchange

Definition
Removal of plasma from the patient and replacement with crystalloid, colloid and protein solutions and/or fresh frozen plasma.

Mechanism of action
Plasma exchange provides means for the almost immediate removal of harmful proteins in the plasma or of substances bound to plasma proteins:

1. paraproteins in hyperviscosity syndrome;
2. antibodies, whether autoantibodies, alloantibodies or isoantibodies (anti-A and anti-B);
3. antigen-antibody complexes;
4. toxic substances, for example thyroxine in 'thyroid storm' or the toxin in mushroom poisoning.

The benefits of plasma exchange depend on the one hand on the distribution of the 'target substance' in the extravascular and intravascular spaces, the rate of equilibration between the two spaces, and the rate of its synthesis, and on the other hand, on the efficiency of removal of the 'target substance' by plasmapheresis, the formation of complexes and their subsequent removal by the mononuclear phagocyte system, and the rate of catabolism. It is important to note that enhanced synthesis of proteins, usually immunoglobulins in myeloma, should be suppressed by administration of immunosuppressive drugs.

Indications

The conditions in which plasma exchange has been beneficial are listed on Table 15.2.

Table 15.2 Diseases and conditions in which plasma exchange has been used as one of the treatment modalities*

Haematological diseases	*Response*
Hyperviscosity syndrome (paraproteinaemia)	excellent
Haemophilia with inhibitors to factor VIII	good
Thrombotic thrombocytopenic purpura	
Immune thrombocytopenic purpura ⎤	good in selected cases
Haemolytic disease of the newborn ⎟	
Autoimmune haemolytic anaemia ⎟	
Bone marrow transplantation ⎦	
Renal diseases	
Goodpasture's syndrome	good
Immune complex glomerulonephritis	good
Renal allograft rejection	uncertain
Neurological diseases	
Myasthenia gravis	good in selected cases
Guillain-Barré syndrome	uncertain
Multiple sclerosis	uncertain
Other disorders	
Fulminant meningococcal septicaemia	good
Familial hypercholesterolaemia	good
Thyroid storm	good
Exogenous intoxication	good
(toxins firmly bound to proteins)	
Systemic lupus erythematosus	uncertain
Rheumatoid arthritis	uncertain

* Number of diseases and conditions in which plasma exchange has been used exceeds 150.

Volume exchanged and replacement fluids

Usually volumes between 2 and 3.5 l of plasma (1 to 1½ volumes of plasma) are exchanged at a time, but it is possible to exchange up to 6 l. Replacement fluids are crystalline solutions such as saline or Ringer's solution, colloid solutions such as dextran, gelatin, plasma protein solution and albumin, or fresh frozen plasma in various proportions. A decision as to the proportions of different replacement solutions used has to be made following assessment of each patient and will take into account the initial level of plasma proteins, the volume of plasma exchanged, frequency of procedures, as well as the effect of the disease and treatment on the concentration of proteins and coagulation factors in the plasma.

Frequency of plasma exchange
Initially plasma exchange can be carried out every day, on alternate days or one or two times weekly. Once the clinical benefit has been achieved plasma exchange can be carried out as maintenance treatment if required.

Adverse reactions are related to
1. establishing the venous access;
2. effect of anticoagulants;
3. effect of replacement fluids, and in particular fresh frozen plasma;
4. loss of normal plasma constituents and the level of their replacement.

Therapeutic leucapheresis

Definition
Removal of leucocytes from the circulation in a patient with raised leucocyte count.

Mechanism of action
Patients with leukaemia with a leucocyte count higher than $150 \times 10^9/l$ may have the hyperviscosity syndrome, or leucostasis, due to disproportionately increased whole blood viscosity. The impaired flow in the microcirculation may give rise to neurological abnormalities, pulmonary dysfunction, thrombotic episodes, priapism and sometimes retinopathy. Leucapheresis will immediately reduce the circulating tumour load and the whole blood viscosity. Following treatment with cytotoxic drugs, leucapheresis may lessen the hazard of hyperuricaemia, hyperphosphataemia and hyperkalaemia.

Indications
The hyperviscosity syndrome in patients with acute myeloid leukaemia or chronic granulocytic leukaemia, whether in chronic phase or blast transformation. In rare instances patients with chronic lymphatic leukaemia may derive some benefit from leucapheresis.

Comment
Good but transient response to leucapheresis has been reported in Sezary's syndrome with a considerable reduction of the size of skin infiltrates, lymph nodes and spleen. Leucapheresis has been used in a few patients with hairy cell leukaemia and prolymphocytic leukaemia prior to splenectomy.
    Note that therapeutic leucapheresis should not be used alone in the treatment of leukaemia, but should be combined with chemotherapy (or splenectomy).

Therapeutic lymphocytapheresis

Therapeutic lymphocytapheresis alone or in combination with plasma exchange has been used for treating rheumatoid arthritis and multiple sclerosis, but convincing evidence for the value of this treatment is still lacking.

Therapeutic platelet apheresis

Therapeutic platelet apheresis may be indicated in patients with essential as well as secondary thrombocythaemia when the platelet count is in excess of $1000 \times 10^9/l$, and when there is a risk of thrombotic or haemorrhagic complications.

Red cell removal and exchange

Definition
Red cell removal, erythrocytapheresis, with or without replacement with donor red cells.

Mechanism of action
Erythrocytapheresis will remove excessive numbers of, or abnormal, red cells from the patient. It has the following advantages over simple blood letting: it is a procedure in which the rate of blood withdrawal and removal of red cells, on the one hand, and infusion of replacement fluids and/or normal red cells, on the other hand, is well balanced. It is, therefore, possible to remove up to 1.7 l of red cells at a time and without replacement or to carry out an exchange transfusion of an adult in one session.

Indications
1. Removal of red cells without replacement (isovolaemic haemodilution) in patients with primary polycythaemia and polycythaemia secondary to chronic obstructive airways disease.
2. Exchange transfusion in adults with sickle cell disease in crisis or preoperatively, and exchange transfusion in patients with fulminant falciparum malaria.

Protocols for erythrocytapheresis are described by manufacturers of blood cell processors and should be adhered to. Autologous plasma is returned to the patient and any deficit in the volume returned is made up by a mixture of crystalloid and colloid solutions and albumin.

The danger of excessive citrate being returned to the patient can be reduced by using
1. heparin instead of a citrate anticoagulant;
2. crystalloid solutions instead of plasma protein fraction, albumin or fresh frozen plasma;
3. packed red cells, washed red cells or frozen and thawed red cells for transfusion.

REFERENCES

Beyer J-H, Klee M, Köstering H, Nagel G A 1980 Coagulation studies before, during and after repeated plasma exchange with 5% human albumin/saline solution in normal donors.

In: Sieberth H G (ed) Plasma exchange. Plasmapheresis-plasmaseparation. Schattaner, Stuttgart

Department of Health and Social Security 1981 A code of practice for automated plasmapheresis of volunteer donors within the UK Blood Transfusion Service

Department of Health and Social Security 1977 A code of practice for the clinical use of blood cell separators

Kennedy M S, Domen R E 1983 Therapeutic apheresis. Applications and future directions. Vox Sanguinis 45: 261–277

Mehta A B, Goldman J M, Kohner E 1984 Hyperleucocytic retinopathy in chronic granulocytic leukaemia: the role of intensive leucapheresis. British Journal of Haematology 56: 661–667

Shumak K H, Rock G A 1984 Therapeutic plasma exchange. New England Journal of Medicine 310: 762–771

16. BLOOD TRANSFUSION IN TRANSPLANTATION

Transfusion of blood and blood components to recipients of kidney or bone marrow transplants may profoundly affect the outcome of transplantation. Thus, general recommendations as well as detailed instructions on blood transfusion are essential in the local transplantation protocol used by specialised units performing these transplantations. By contrast, blood transfusion has little effect on the outcome of transplantation of the liver, pancreas and heart. In this chapter only the main issues of transplantation pertinent to transfusion of blood and blood components are presented.

KIDNEY TRANSPLANTATION

Need for transfusion
Prospective recipients of kidney transplants may require blood transfusion for alleviating severe anaemia either present during the course of their illness or immediately prior to and during the operation. It is unusual for these patients to require support with other blood components and products.

Effect of transfusion on graft survival
Contrary to earlier belief there is now little doubt that blood transfusions have a beneficial effect on cadaver kidney graft survival. However two major issues, the mechanisms involved and the risk of sensitisation, still remain controversial. In spite of that, a number of transplantation protocols currently in use incorporate blood transfusion even to those prospective recipients who do not require blood for correction of anaemia. Further data are needed to establish the value of the volume of blood transfused, the freshness and leucocyte content of blood, number of transfusions and the interval between them, etc.

A patient who has received a kidney from a related donor, and has also received donor-specific transfusions (DST) prior to transplantation, has a considerably better chance of having a prolonged kidney graft survival. Using DST it is also possible to segregate the responders to immunogenic stimulation from non-responders by careful monitoring of specific humoral responses to the donor's antigens. As only non-responders proceed to transplantation the early rejection of the graft is avoided. *Note* that the recipients of DST should not be transfused with blood or blood components from a third party.

Mechanism of action

Repetitive transfusions of donor-specific antigens in a modest dose may induce some degree of specific non-responsiveness to the same antigens present on the subsequently transplanted kidney. Other mechanisms most likely involved in prolonging the graft survival depend on the production of antibodies such as those against recognition sites on T lymphocytes or against alloantibodies, for example anti-Fab and anti-IgG antibodies. The overall effect is a suppression of the immune response of the kidney recipient. There is also evidence that repeated blood transfusions may affect phagocytosis by mononuclear cells and thus by non-specific immunosuppression prolong graft survival.

Alloimmunisation

As the number of transfusions increases, the proportion of patients with no detectable antibodies decreases. However, the rate of sensitisation by multiple transfusions is relatively low. In one group of patients 40% of those who received more than 11 transfusions developed antibodies but only 15% developed high levels. Also, genetic factors may be implicated in the strength of immunological response, since patients homozygous for HLA-DR3 appear to have a particularly low responsiveness to histocompatibility antigens.

Cytomegalovirus infection may have serious consequences for kidney recipients. Therefore, when both the kidney donor and recipient are anti-CMV negative, the recipient should be transfused with blood and blood components collected from anti-CMV negative donors. Logically, that recommendation should be extended to blood and blood components used for transfusion of all anti-CMV negative potential kidney graft recipients.

Plasma exchange used for decreasing the concentration of antibodies responsible for acute rejection of the kidney graft has not yet been proved to be of benefit.

BONE MARROW TRANSPLANTATION

Bone marrow transplantation has become an accepted method of treating marrow failure in aplastic anaemia, acute leukaemia and chronic granulocytic leukaemia as well as in some non-haematological disorders. The relationship between blood transfusion and some aspects of marrow transplantation, e.g. graft rejection, graft versus host disease, prevention and treatment of haemorrhage and infections of bacterial and viral origin, will be discussed below.

Need for transfusion and selection of donors

Recipients of bone marrow are likely to require transfusion before transplantation, and they will invariably require it during the period of marrow engraftment.

1. *Before transplantation* Patients with *aplastic anaemia* and all
   the family members should be HLA typed as soon as possible
   following the diagnosis. If an HLA identical member of the
   family, capable of and willing to donate bone marrow, is
   identified, early transplantation is the treatment of choice,
   and transfusion of blood and blood components, if required,
   should be given from random donors only. Transfusion from
   family members should be avoided under all circumstances.
   Similarly patients with *leukaemia* should be transfused with
   blood and blood components collected from random donors,
   and transfusion from family members should be avoided.

2. *After bone marrow transplantation* patients with aplastic
   anaemia and with leukaemia will require intensive transfusion
   support during the four to six week period of engraftment.
   The requirements for blood will vary considerably between
   individual patients (Fig. 16.1).

   Platelet concentrates from random donors should be given
   until the patient becomes refractory; HLA typed or
   cross-matched platelet concentrates will then be required
   (p. 58). Ideal support is provided by plateletpheresing the
   marrow donor. For patients with aplastic anaemia, platelets

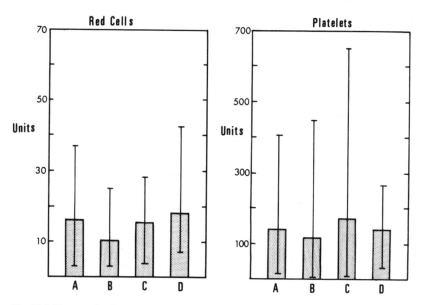

Fig. 16.1 The use of red cells and platelet concentrates in patients with aplastic anaemia and leukaemia following bone marrow transplantation. The mean number of units and range per patient are represented by columns and vertical bars, respectively. A: 20 patients with aplastic anaemia; B: 20 patients with acute leukaemia in remission; C: 20 patients with acute leukaemia in relapse; D: 12 patients with chronic myelogenous leukaemia (3 patients in the chronic phase, 2 patients in 'accelerated' phase and 7 patients in blast crisis). (The illustration is based on data by Storb R and Weiden P L, 1981)

from family members can be given one to two days before the first dose of cyclophosphamide. In patients receiving total body irradiation, platelets from family members should not be given until after irradiation.

Patients with neutropenia and severe infection resistant to treatment with antibiotics will require granulocyte concentrates, which are preferred to buffy coats. A single donor, ideally the marrow donor, or another relative sharing at least one HLA haplotype, should be leucapheresed.

Irradiation of blood and blood components
All units of blood and all blood components to be used for transfusion to recipients of bone marrow grafts must be irradiated with a dose of 1500 to 3000 rads (15 to 30 Gy) to prevent immunocompetent cells from engrafting, and producing graft versus host disease.

Cytomegalovirus infection is one of the serious complications of bone marrow transplantation (p. 116). When both the donor and the recipient of the graft are anti-CMV negative, blood and blood components collected from anti-CMV negative donors should be used. Trials to establish the value of anti-CMV immunoglobulin in the prevention and treatment of CMV infection are in progress.

ABO incompatible bone marrow transplantation is associated with two potential complications:

1. An acute haemolytic transfusion reaction at the time of bone marrow transfusion (for example, when the donor is group A or B and recipient group O). It can be prevented by (a) removal of antibodies in the recipient by plasma exchange or by solid phase immunoadsorbent columns with A or B substance, (b) removal of red cells from the bone marrow graft using centrifugation and washing in a blood cell processor.
2. Persistent haemolysis following transplantation caused by the host's anti-A or-B antibodies. Most of the patients have a positive DAT and detectable antibodies in the serum, which gradually disappear as the production of antibodies ceases. If transfusion with blood is required, group O red cells should be administered.

Albumin (albumin solution and plasma protein fraction) may be required during the recovery phase of marrow transplantation as an adjuvant to parenteral nutrition. Albumin is used empirically and no guidelines for its use exist at present.

TRANSPLANTATION OF OTHER ORGANS

Transfusion of blood and blood components to recipients of liver, pancreas or heart transplants does not appear to affect the outcome of transplantation. However, in liver transplantation all the problems of massive transfusion are encountered (p. 37) and in some cases the demand for blood and blood components may be very high (initially up to 60 units). It is essential to inform the Regional Transfusion Centre of the forthcoming operation so that a stock of blood can be held in reserve. In addition a sufficient number of units of fresh frozen plasma and platelet concentrates should be available. Heart transplantation does not pose problems other than those associated with open heart surgery (p. 39).

REFERENCES

Storb R, Weiden P L 1981 Transfusion problems associated with transplantation. In: Conrad M E (ed) Transfusion problems in haematology. Seminars in Hematology 18: 163–176
Terasaki P I (ed) 1982 Blood transfusion and transplantation. Grune & Stratton, New York
Woodruff M F A, van Rood J J 1983 Possible implications of the effect of blood transfusion on allograft survival. Lancet 1: 1201–1203

17. ORGANISATION OF BLOOD TRANSFUSION IN A MAJOR ACCIDENT

In a major accident numbers of people may be injured within a short space of time by mechanical forces, chemicals, fire or fumes. The rescue of live casualities and provision of treatment require a coordinated action of the Ambulance Service, Fire Brigade and Police on the one hand, and the hospital designated for admission of casualties on the other hand. A plan of action, 'Major Accident Procedure', is therefore prepared by every hospital so designated, and it should be periodically tested by holding a 'major accident exercise'. All heads of department are expected to be familiar with the action required of the department in the event of a major accident. The following aspects of preparation for a major accident are related to the work undertaken by the blood bank.

Information that a disaster has occurred will be first accepted by the Emergency Service. The nearest designated hospital will immediately be informed. On receiving the call, the hospital switchboard operator will immediately implement instructions for action and will telephone all the individuals (or departments) on the 'need to know' list, which will include the blood bank and the consultant in charge. The most senior member of the staff in the blood bank will then implement existing instructions for action.

Role of the blood bank
The main objectives of the blood bank are to ensure that the necessary stock of blood and blood products, judged by information received regarding the nature of the accident and estimated number of casualties, is maintained throughout the emergency, and to ensure that the policy for issuing blood is implemented.

The first objective is achieved by suspending the issue of blood for non-emergency transfusions and by increasing the stock to the desired level by arranging delivery(ies) from the nearest hospital and/or Regional Transfusion Centre. The blood bank must therefore have an outside telephone line because the switchboard will be flooded by incoming calls.

The policy for issuing blood for transfusion in a major disaster is the same as that used for emergency transfusions (p. 187). Compatibility testing should be carried out whenever possible. If that is not possible every attempt should be made to determine the ABO and Rh groups so that group specific or compatible blood can be issued. When the recipient's blood group is not known, group O Rh positive blood is used for transfusion to boys and men; group O Rh negative blood should be given to girls and women in the reproductive age, except when a life threatening haemorrhage requires transfusion and O Rh-negative blood is not available. Blood products are usually not required in large amounts, but an ample stock of fresh frozen plasma should be available as well as some platelet concentrates for those patients who are receiving massive transfusions. PPF should be reserved for treating patients with burns.

In the pressure of an emergency, special care must be taken in the identification of casualties, and in labelling samples of blood, reports and cross-matched units of blood; at least the record number and sex of the recipient must be known. Since this is a part of the procedures planned in advance every member of staff should be familiar with its implementation.

Organisation of a blood donors' clinic

Following a major accident relatives and friends of the casualties, as well as members of the public at large may wish to donate blood. It is unlikely that the hospital admitting the casualties could provide medical and nursing staff to man a donor clinic. Therefore, potential donors should be advised to attend at the nearest Regional Transfusion Centre on that day or return to the hospital on the following day, when the team from the Regional Transfusion Centre will hold a donor clinic. That information should be made available to those inquiring by telephone, it should be prominently displayed on posters, and when necessary released to the public information media (press, local radio station).

18. PROCEDURES FOR TRANSFUSION OF BLOOD AND BLOOD COMPONENTS

The main role of a hospital blood transfusion laboratory (the blood bank) is to provide compatible blood for transfusion to patients. To achieve this the blood bank keeps an inventory of blood and blood products and performs basic immunohaematological tests. The blood and blood components are supplied by the Regional Blood Transfusion Centre, although in some countries the blood bank may also be responsible wholly or in part for donor recruitment and the collection of blood. Hospital blood banks often have links with centres or institutions to which they can refer samples for complex and technically difficult testing.

Although the organisation of work may vary from one blood bank to another, similar steps are required to ensure that compatible blood is administered to the patient. These steps are the generation of the request, collection of blood sample from the patient, immunohaematological testing, and reporting and record keeping.

DECISION TO TRANSFUSE

Red cell replacement
In *acute blood loss*, clinical assessment of the patient and the measurement of blood loss (when possible) are a better guide than haemoglobin concentration or haematocrit. In *chronic anaemia* transfusion should be used only if the patient has failed to respond or is unlikely to respond to specific therapy (iron, folic acid or vitamin B_{12}); also if the patient's clinical condition (myocardial infarction, cerebrovascular accident, severe infection) makes transfusion imperative. In *transfusion dependent patients* the time of transfusion and the amount of blood given are known in advance and the transfusion is often arranged to suit the patient and the blood bank.

Platelets
Platelet transfusions are given to either arrest or prevent bleeding in a severely thrombocytopenic patient or in a patient whose platelets are functionally abnormal.

Fresh frozen plasma
Fresh frozen plasma is administered when non-specific haemostatic replacement is required, e.g. after massive transfusion, in DIC, after

cardiopulmonary bypass, in liver disease, rapid anticoagulant reversal, etc.

Factor VIII preparations and other clotting factor concentrates

Factor VIII concentrates and cryoprecipitate are administered to prevent or arrest bleeding in haemophiliacs. Other concentrates are used in specific factor deficiencies.

Plasma protein fraction and albumin

PPF and albumin are used as volume expanders in a variety of situations. Albumin is also given to replace excessive loss of albumin in acute liver disease, acute nephrotic syndrome, burns, etc.

Choice of blood or blood component

Red cells

Whole blood, plasma reduced blood or packed cells can be given to replace acute blood loss. In chronic anaemia, packed cells or plasma reduced blood should always be chosen. White cell depleted blood is required for patients with a previous history of febrile reactions to blood.

Platelets

In an emergency or for an individual who is receiving platelets for the first time, random donor platelets are used. For those on long term prophylactic platelet transfusions who become refractory, HLA matched cell separator platelets are subsequently required.

Factor VIII

In an emergency either cryoprecipitate or factor VIII concentrate can be given. For those requiring high doses of factor VIII, concentrate preparations are recommended. Small children should preferably receive cryoprecipitate in order to minimize the risk of hepatitis and AIDS.

Amount to be transfused

Red cells

In an adult (60–70 kg) who is not bleeding, each unit of blood (200 ml of red cells) raises the haemoglobin concentration on average by 1 g/dl and the PCV by 0.03 l/l. In a patient who is actively bleeding at the time of transfusion, the response cannot be assessed by blood count: accurate assessment is made by monitoring the CVP. If this is not possible, clinical observation (e.g. a warm periphery, systolic blood pressure over 70 mm Hg etc) is the only guide.

In children with anaemia the rule of thumb for estimating the amount of blood needed is:

$$V = (PCV_1 - PCV_0) \times BW$$

where V is the volume of red cells to be transfused in ml, PCV_1 and PCV_0 are the desired and the initial PCV, and BW is the body weight in kg. Remember that each unit contains on average 200 ml red cells.

Blood ordering for surgery

An ordering policy for cross-matching prior to surgery is essential, since it is time consuming and costly to cross-match blood for surgical interventions which rarely if ever require blood transfusion. 'Group and save serum' is adequate for the surgical interventions listed in Table 18.1, unless there is a specific reason (anaemia, history of previous bleeding, liver disease, known disorder of haemostasis) why a full cross-match should be done. A 'group and save' policy is even safer if it is run as a 'group and screen' (i.e. antibody screen) policy: all patients would thus be checked for irregular antibodies prior to surgery. The usual amount of blood required for surgical operations invariably using blood is shown in Table 18.2. This is a rough guide only and special procedures and individual needs (of both surgeons and patients) must be taken into account.

Table 18.1 Some surgical procedures for which 'group and save' policy is safe*

General surgery	Orthopaedic surgery
Cholecystectomy	Removal of pin & plate
Laparotomy	Excision of intervertebral disk
Vagotomy and pyloroplasty	Limb amputation for ischaemic disease
Partial gastrectomy	Meniscectomy
Construction of ileostomy	Osteotomy
Haemorrhoidectomy	
Hernia repair	
Simple mastectomy	
Thyroidectomy	
Gynaecology	Neurosurgery
Abdominal hysterectomy	Laminectomy
Vaginal hysterectomy	Trephine and burr-hole biopsy
Repair of prolapse	
Ovarian cystectomy	Urology
D & C	Cystoscopy
	TUR of a bladder lesion
Vascular surgery	
Vein stripping	

* Unless the patient has a known bleeding tendency or there are other reasons to believe that he or she may bleed excessively

Table 18.2 Number of units of blood usually required in some common surgical procedures

General surgery	Units	Orthopaedics	Units
Splenectomy	2	Spinal fusion	3
Bowel resection	3	Total hip replacement	3
Total gastrectomy	3	Total knee replacement	3
Pancreatectomy	4	Pin and plate for fractured neck	2
Abdominoperineal resection	4	of femur	
Oesophagectomy	4		
Neurosurgery		Urology	
Carrotid endarterectomy	4	Partial cystectomy	2
Craniotomy	2	Total cystectomy	4
		Nephrectomy	2
Obstetrics		Nephrolithotomy	2
LSCS	2	Prostatectomy (open)	2
		Prostatectomy (TUR)	2

Platelets

Six to eight single donor units or one cell separator unit is required to raise an adult recipient's platelet count by $10 \times 10^9/l$, if he is not bleeding, not infected, has no antiplatelet antibodies and no splenomegaly.

Fresh frozen plasma

5–15 ml per kg body weight is given as haemostatic replacement.

Factor VIII

The dose of factor VIII varies according to body weight and to the nature of haemorrhage. For small spontaneous joint bleeds 15–20 i.u./kg are usually enough, whereas for severe haemarthroses, haematomata or to cover operations, much larger doses (up to 100 i.u./kg) are administered.

Plasma protein fraction, and albumin

500–2000 ml of PPF is given daily depending on the patient's condition. 20% albumin is administered in doses of 2–6 ml/kg body weight/24 hrs.

Collection of blood for laboratory testing

Request form

The collection of a blood sample is initiated by the clinician who is personally responsible for completing and signing a request form. The information required on the form is necessary for the identification of the patient, to provide his medical and transfusion history and to state the reason for requesting blood for transfusion and/or a particular investigation (Table 18.3). It is desirable to state on the form the degree

Table 18.3 Information which should be available when immunohaematological tests and/or blood and blood components for transfusion are requested

Identification of the patient:
    Surname
    First names
    Sex
    Date of birth
    Hospital record number
    Ward
    Name of consultant in charge
    Name of doctor requesting the test
Medical and transfusion history:
    Blood group, if previously determined
    Number of pregnancies (for women)
    Previous transfusions of blood and blood products
    Previous transfusion reactions
    Presence of antibodies against red cells, if previously demonstrated
    Date of last transfusion
Reasons for request:
    Medical diagnosis
    Reasons for the tests
    Tests requested
When blood or blood components are requested:
    Number of units
    Date and time when blood or blood components should be available

of urgency and the expected time by which the report and/or blood should be available.

Identification of the patient must be carried out both by questioning the conscious patient and by matching the name and hospital registration number on the request form with that on the identity wrist band. Errors of identification of the patient (or the blood sample) account for the majority of transfusion 'disasters' and they are legally indefensible.

Collection of blood

A volume of venous blood sufficient for the tests requested (Table 18.4) is withdrawn usually from an anticubital vein. In babies and children blood may be obtained by heelpricks and fingerpricks and can be used satisfactorily for blood grouping and compatibility testing. The neonate is grouped on cord blood, blood obtained from a heelprick or from venepuncture, but the compatibility tests are carried out using mother's serum (see p. 35). Blood from drains, administration sets and body cavities is unsuitable for blood grouping and compatibility testing.

Identification of the blood sample

The container(s) must be carefully labelled and dated *after* being filled with blood. On receiving samples and request forms, the blood bank will discard all incompletely or illegibly filled forms, samples with incompletely and illegibly filled labels and samples where the identification on the label does not match that on the request form.

Table 18.4 Basic immunohaematological investigations carried out by a blood bank and the volume of blood required

	Volume of blood required	
Investigation	Plain tube, ml	EDTA* tube, ml
Blood group determination	5	None**
Compatibility testing	10	(5)
Antibody screening and identification	20	5
Red cell phenotype determination	20	5
Antiglobulin test, direct and indirect	5	5
Detection of cold agglutinins	10†	5

* Sodium or potassium salt of EDTA
** It is possible to determine the blood group using 5 ml of blood collected into an EDTA tube.
† Blood must be collected using a warm syringe and needle, the sample held, and the serum separated from the red cells at 37°C.

Collection of blood from blood bank

Units of compatibility tested blood awaiting collection are kept in a separate refrigerator in the blood bank. They are issued by the laboratory staff or, out of hours, collected by designated persons. The person collecting blood must carry the documentation which specifies the patient's details as well as the information regarding the unit(s) of blood, and must check that identification details relating to the patient and to the unit agree, make record of issue in the issue book, and sign it.

The compatibility label on the unit of blood should contain the patient's first name(s) and surname, hospital number, blood group, number of the unit and the date of transfusion, as requested. When there is any discrepancy between the documentation and the compatibility label the unit is not issued (or collected).

Ward procedure

The ward procedure for transfusion of blood, blood components and blood products must be clearly defined and agreed between nursing and medical staff.

The unit of blood should be checked at the bedside by two people, one of whom is either a state registered nurse or a doctor. The patient should be asked his name and the information compared with that on his identification bracelet, on the compatibility label and on the compatibility report in the patient's notes. At the same time the ABO and Rh group of the unit should be checked with that on the blood group report and the compatibility label. The expiry date of the unit is checked, and the unit firmly squeezed to test for leaks.

Unconscious patient must be identified by the wrist band. Patients without identification shoul not be transfused except in dire emergency. If this is the case, the doctor in charge must make the best identification possible, record his action in the notes and only then proceed with transfusion.

For each unit of blood transfused, its number, date of transfusion and the starting and finishing time should be recorded on a special intravenous administration form, and the person who checked the details of the unit and connected it should sign the record. This form is permanently retained in the patient's notes.

For the procedure followed in the case of a transfusion reaction see p. 92.

Blood components which have the unique donation number, e.g. platelet and granulocyte concentrates, fresh frozen plasma and cryoprecipitate, are collected and checked in the same way as the blood.

Blood products which have a batch number, e.g. coagulation factor concentrates, albumin solution and immunoglobulins, may be collected either from the blood bank or from the pharmacy, depending on local arrangements. The procedure followed for collection and administration of blood products is that used for all intravenous fluids in the hospital. Careful recording of batch numbers is essential for the inquiry following an untoward reaction or transmission of a disease.

Premedication of the recipient

In *acute blood loss* no premedication is required since the primary concern is to replace the volume lost and establish an adequate oxygen supply to the tissues. Patients with *chronic anaemia* are given a fast acting diuretic (such as frusemide, 20 to 40 mg i.v.) prior to each unit of blood to diminish the effect of transfusion on the circulatory volume. Recipients with a history of a previous non-haemolytic febrile transfusion reaction or anaphylactoid reactions or those receiving granulocyte concentrates should be given hydrocortisone, 100 mg i.v. as well as an antihistamine (chlorpheniramine, Piriton, 10 mg) orally or intravenously.

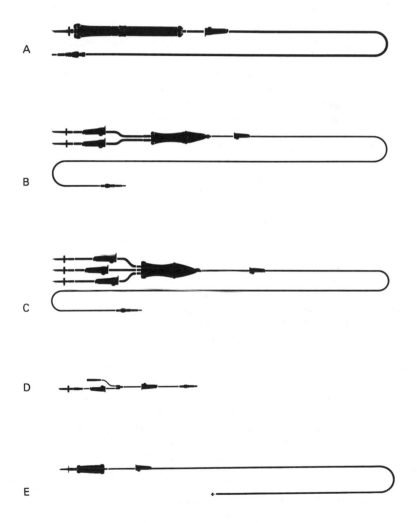

Fig. 18.1 Blood administration sets and equipment. Sets illustrated are manufactured by Travenol Laboratories Limited and similar sets are available from several other manufacturers. (a) administration set for blood and blood derivatives; (b) Y-type administration set; (c) triple-lead plasmapheresis set; (d) cryoprecipitate and platelet administration set; (e) platelet administration set. (Reproduced from: Blood Administration Sets. Specifications and configurations. With kind permission of Travenol Laboratories Limited)

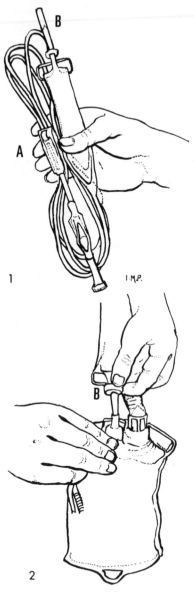

Fig. 18.2 Preparation for transfusion using an administration set for blood and blood derivatives. (1) Close clamp (A). (2) Mix blood thoroughly; pull tabs on the pack to expose outlet post. Remove coupler cover (B) and insert into outlet with twisting motion. (3) Remove protective cover from needle adapter (C), open clamp (D). Hold blood pack inverted, squeeze blood to fill filter chamber (E) completely and drip chamber (F) to about a quarter. Close clamp (D). (4) Suspend blood pack. (5) Attach needle to the adaptor (C), open clamp (D), allow blood to fill the set and expel the air. Close clamp (D). You are now ready to perform the venepuncture or to attach the needle adapter to the butterfly already sited in the vein. (Redrawn from: Transfusion with the straight type blood recipient set and blood-pack unit, Fenwal E 239–2/79, with kind permission of Travenol Laboratories Limited)

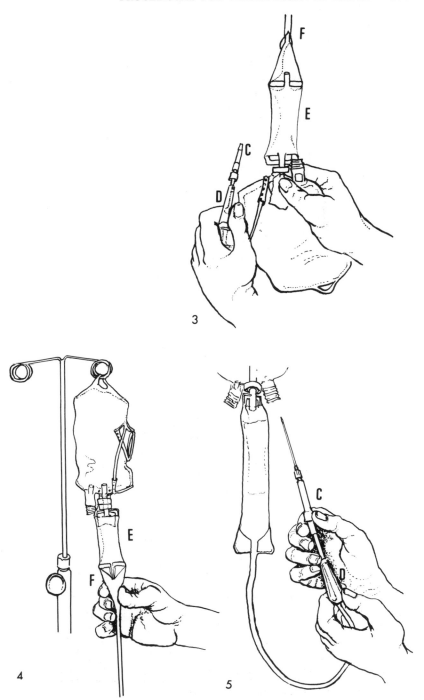

3

4   5

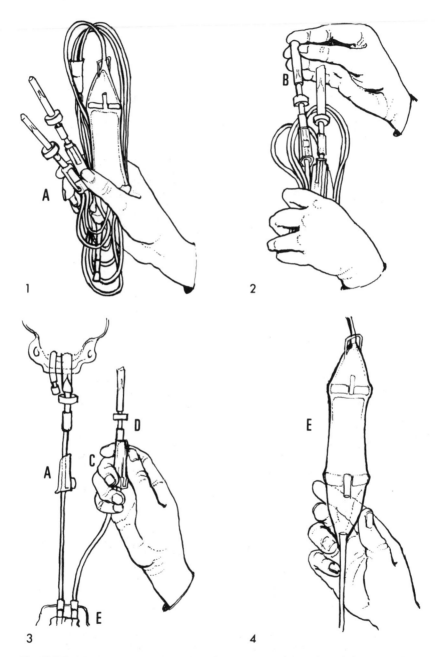

Fig. 18.3 Preparation for transfusion using a Y-type administration set for blood and blood derivatives. (1) Close clamp (A). (2) Remove one coupler cover (B), insert coupler into the pack containing solution and suspend container. (3) Open clamp (A) on the lead below solution. Open clamp (C) on the adjacent lead. Close clamp (A) when chamber (E) is full. (4) Squeeze and release drip chamber (E) until one quarter filled.

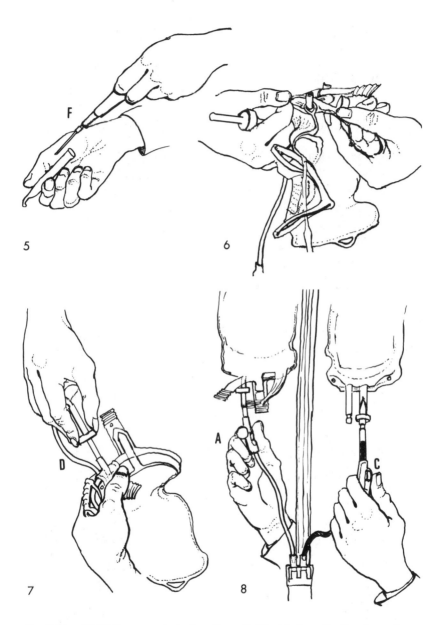

Fig. 18.3 (cont'd) (5) Remove protector from the needle (F). Attach needle. Open lower clamp (see Fig. 18.2) to fill with solution and expel air. Perform venepuncture. (6) Mix blood in the pack. Close all clamps. Pull apart tabs to expose outlet port. (7) Remove coupler cover (D) from unused lead; insert into outlet port; suspend blood pack. (8) Close clamp (A) under saline container; open clamp (C) under blood pack. Open lower clamp and adjust flow rate. (Redrawn from: Transfusion with Y-type blood-solution recipient set and blood-pack unit, Fenwal, E 238-2/79, with kind permission of Travenol Laboratories Limited)

Setting up the transfusion

Before bringing the blood or blood component to the bedside it is necessary to prepare the stand and holders for blood packs or bottles, and the administration sets (also called recipient or giving sets) for the transfusion.

Blood and red cells

A straight recipient set or 'Y' recipient set, is used (Fig. 18.1). The procedure of connecting the set to a pack of sterile saline is shown in Fig. 18.2 and 18.3.

Platelets, cryoprecipitate and factor VIII concentrate

A platelet recipient set or platelet cryoprecipitate recipient set is required (Fig. 18.1). The procedure of connecting these sets to the unit of platelets and to pooled cryoprecipitate is shown in Fig. 18.2.

Factor VIII concentrate is a freeze-dried preparation which is reconstituted with the specified volume of sterile water, taken up into a syringe (60 ml) and injected directly into the vein. Small quantities of cryoprecipitate can also be pooled in the syringe and injected directly. A butterfly needle facilitates the handling of a large syringe.

Fresh frozen plasma is administered through a straight recipient set.

PPF and albumin are solutions in glass bottles. They are also infused using a straight recipient set with an airway (see Fig. 18.2).

Site of transfusion

The best sites are the veins of the dorsum of the hand and on the forearm. If no veins of sufficient calibre are available in these sites use the antecubital vein. It is less convenient for the patient because an arm splint will be required to immobilize the elbow joint in extension. In infants a scalp vein may have to be used. Use veins on the lower limb and other sites only if there are no accessible veins on the arms.

Scrub hands thoroughly and prepare the skin site meticulously. When transfusing immunosuppressed or neutropenic patients use sterile gloves and a sterile field technique.

Needles and catheters

Needles and catheters from size 14 to size 20 are used. The largest size suitable for the calibre of the vein is selected. In adults sizes 16, 17 and 18 are preferred. In children 18, 19 or 20 are usually required.

Once the appropriate needle or catheter is in the vein connect it to the recipient set, which should be already attached to the unit of blood or to the required blood product.

Use of filters

All recipient sets contain a standard 170 µm filter and are used to remove the largest microaggregates which form in stored blood. Microaggregate filters may be used to remove all microaggregates over the size of 20 μm. Never use leukocyte or microaggregate filters when giving cryoprecipitate, platelet or granulocyte concentrates.

Temperature of blood

Cold blood may be dangerous for recipients since it may provoke cardiac arrythmias and even asystole. Always ensure that the blood is warmed up to at least room temperature before transfusing it. If large quantities of blood are to be given quickly the blood should be warmed up to body temperature in a water bath. In an emergency, blood may have to be taken from the refrigerator and virtually immediately transfused. In this case *always* use an in-line blood warmer. Always check the temperature as overheating may cause haemolysis with severe transfusion reaction.

Rate of infusion

The rate of infusion must be decided in advance. Standard giving sets are calibrated to deliver 1 ml of blood in about 15 drops. In acute blood loss, blood is given at rates of up to 100 ml/min until systolic blood pressure reaches 100 mm Hg. For rates higher than this, sometimes needed in severe arterial haemorrhage, special devices for ensuring rapid transfusion must be used. Packed cells and plasma reduced blood have too high a viscosity to allow such rapid transfusion rates. The rate can be increased by reducing the haematocrit of the unit transfused: this is achieved by mixing red cells and sterile isotonic saline using a 'Y' recipient set. 50 to 100 ml saline is usually added per unit of red cells.

In chronic anaemia never exceed a rate of 2 ml/min (four hours for each unit of whole blood). Recipients with cardiac, respiratory or renal disease must always be transfused cautiously; when more than two units of blood are required it is safer to give the transfusion on two separate days.

Note that the only solution that can be safely mixed with blood is sterile physiological saline. Dextrose solutions may cause osmotic lysis and/or aggregation of red cells in the tubing. Ringer's lactate contains ionized calcium and may provoke fibrin formation in the tubing with subsequent blockage.

Platelet transfusions are given one pack at time, six to eight units per one to two hours. Cryoprecipitate and factor VIII concentrate are administered at a rate not exceeding 10 ml/min. The rate of transfusion of plasma protein fraction and albumin depends on the circulatory state of the recipient.

Monitoring the patient

The patient should be watched closely during the first 30 min of transfusion to see that the desired rate of infusion is maintained and to observe whether any untoward reactions occur. In acute blood loss, especially if due to a severe injury, monitoring is part of intensive resuscitation. It generally includes observation of the CVP, as well as measurement of pulse rate, blood pressure, respiratory rate and urinary output. As already mentioned, CVP monitoring, patient observation and assessment of blood loss are more important indicators of the patient's condition than blood counts.

In the less acute situation, the patient should be made warm and comfortable in an upright position. After the first half an hour of intensive observation half-hourly pulse rate, temperature and blood pressure are recorded. In special situations, e.g. patients with severe anaemia or history of transfusion reaction, more detailed and more frequent observations may be necessary. In particular, during platelet or clotting factor infusions, check the patient frequently for febrile and anaphylactic reactions. Slow down or discontinue the infusion if any untoward effects are observed. Always keep the i.v. line open with a small amount of sterile saline.

The transfusion site should be easily accessible and preferably visible through a transparent dressing so that any extravasation, inflammation or 'bogginess'can immediately be seen.

Final check-up

When the transfusion is completed, remove the needle, check that the site shows no inflammation, apply pressure to arrest bleeding and cover with a sterile dressing. If the site is red, hot and tender, send the catheter tip or the fluid obtained by rinsing it with sterile saline for bacteriological tests. Patients at risk from circulatory overload should be observed from 12 to 24 hours after transfusion (see p. 102). Return all empty blood packs to the blood bank which will keep them for 48 hours before disposal (after 48 hours the occurrence of a transfusion reaction which may require tests on these units is unlikely).

REFERENCES

BSCH Blood Group and Transfusion Task Force 1984 Guide lines on hospital blood bank documentation and procedures. The British Society for Haematology
Department of Health and Social Security 1984 Notes on transfusion
Smallwood J A 1983 Use of blood in elective general surgery: an area of wasted resources. British Medical Journal 286: 868–870

19. BASIC IMMUNO-HAEMATOLOGICAL METHODS AND RECORD KEEPING

IMMUNOHAEMATOLOGICAL METHODS

Principles

Immunohaematological reactions are based on the interaction between an antigen and the corresponding antibody. The reaction between red cell antigens and their antibodies is described below and that between platelet, granulocyte and plasma protein antigens and their antibodies in Chapter 4.

The end result of red cell antigen-antibody reaction in vitro is agglutination which can be seen by eye or microscopically; rarely the end result is haemolysis. The reaction occurs in two stages, in the first stage the antibody is bound to the red cell, and in the second stage the agglutination occurs.

Factors affecting *the first stage* of the antigen-antibody reaction are:

1. Physico-chemical properties of the antibody which determine the binding constant; thus an antibody may be 'strongly' or 'weakly' bound to the red cell.

2. The optimum binding temperature: IgM molecules (cold antibodies) generally bind to the red cell best at 4°C, whereas the binding of IgG molecules (warm antibodies) is most efficient at 37°C.

3. The ionic strength of the suspension medium: low ionic strength increases the rate of binding. This is the basis for tests using low ioning strength saline (LISS).

4. The optimum pH for binding: outside the pH range from 4 to 9 the binding of antibodies to antigens usually does not occur.

Factors affecting *the second stage* of the antigen-antibody reaction bring about agglutination by overcoming the repellent force of negatively charged red cells suspended in saline (zeta potential). The size of the IgM molecule (complete antibody) is sufficient to bridge the gap between two red cells and thus enable agglutination to occur, but the IgG molecule (incomplete antibody) is too small to do so unless the electric charge is reduced or overcome by one of the following means:

1. The proximity of antibody-coated cells can be increased by centrifugation at low speed ('spin' techniques).

2. The contact between cells is also improved in the presence of albumin, probably due to an alteration in the electric charge.
3. The electric charge of the red cell can be reduced by incubating red cells with papain, trypsin, bromelin or ficin (enzyme treatment).
4. The agglutination of red cells coated with an IgG (incomplete) antibody, as well as an IgA antibody or complement, may be brought about by addition of anti-immunoglobulin serum. The reaction is the basis of the direct and indirect antiglobulin tests described later.

Tests

Basic immunohaematological investigations carried out by the blood bank are listed in Table 18.4. A fresh sample of venous blood is required.

Blood group determination

Definition
Determination of the ABO and Rh(D) groups.
Indications
Prospective recipients of transfusion of blood or blood components, pregnant women, workers in dangerous occupations, participants in dangerous sports, members of the armed forces, blood donors.
Principles of the ABO group determination
The person's red cells are tested using antisera which contain potent IgM saline agglutinating anti-A, anti-B and anti-A,B antibodies, and the serum is tested using known group A, B and O red cells (reverse blood grouping).
Potential problems in ABO grouping
1. Red cells of A and B subgroups are weakly agglutinated, the agglutination may be missed and the blood wrongly grouped.
2. The conflicting finding of the simultaneous presence of A or B antigen on the red cells and the corresponding antibody in the serum may be due to (a) acquired A or B antigen, (b) alteration of red cell antigens by bacterial enzymes in a contaminated sample of blood, and (c) presence of autoantibodies.
3. Interpretation of agglutination may be difficult in the presence of high concentration of paraproteins in the serum and when the sample of blood was taken following administration of high molecular weight dextran, because apparent agglutination is seen in all tubes.
4. The recent administration of compatible but not group specific blood such as group O to a group A or AB recipient is usually easily recognised by 'mixed field' agglutination.

Principle of the Rh(D) grouping
Red cells are tested using an antiserum containing an IgM sufficiently potent to agglutinate Rh(D)-positive cells in saline. Further tests to detect D^u antigen using an IgG antibody and the antiglobulin test are carried out in some blood banks only on Rh(D)-negative samples and in other blood banks on all samples. All pregnant women and blood donors should be tested for D^u.

A potential problem in Rh(D) grouping is a weak agglutination, usually due to D^u or D variants, which may be missed. The importance of distinguishing Rh(D)-negative from Rh(D^u)-positive individuals is discussed on p. 13.

Compatibility testing

Definition
In vitro demonstration of serological compatibility between the prospective recipient's (patient's) serum and donor's red cells.

The aim is the prevention of haemolytic transfusion reaction caused by the administration of incompatible blood. Compatibility testing should be carried out within the 48 hours before administration of blood to the patient. Only exceptionally may blood for transfusion be issued without compatibility testing (see below).

Group specific blood
1. Blood of the same ABO group as that of the prospective recipient, is selected for transfusion. When group specific blood is unavailable, blood of other groups may be selected provided that it is compatible (Table 19.1).
2. In general Rh(D)-positive recipients should receive Rh(D)-positive blood and Rh(D)-negative recipients must receive Rh(D)-negative blood. If supplies are limited, the decision to transfuse a Rh(D)-negative recipient with Rh(D)-positive blood must be made after assessing each case individually;

Table 19.1 Selection of blood for transfusion according to the patient's ABO group

Patient's blood group	Blood for transfusion	
	Blood group, first choice	Blood group when the first choice is not available*
O	O	—
A	A	O
A_2 with anti-A_1	A_2	O
B	B	O
AB	AB	A or B (exceptionally O)
A_2B with anti-A_1	A_2B	A_2 or B (exceptionally O)

* It is advisable to use red cell concentrate or plasma reduced blood unless the clinical situation makes the transfusion of whole blood essential.

but Rh(D)-positive blood must never be given to Rh(D)-negative girls and women in the reporudctive age. Recipients with proven D^u antigen need not receive Rh(D)-negative blood (see p. 14).

Principle of the technique
Compatibility is tested by incubating recipient's serum and donor's red cells (the major cross-match). As a control, recipient's own serum and red cells are also incubated. The absence of agglutination in both tests indicates that a gross error in the ABO grouping of the recipient and donor has not been made, and that the presence of allo- or autoantibodies in the recipient's serum is unlikely, and therefore, that the blood tested is safe for transfusion. The donor's cells may be prepared in several ways for presentation to the recipient's serum and a combination of the following methods is generally used:

(a) the red cells may be suspended in saline at room temperature,

(b) the cells may be suspended in albumin or in low ionic strength saline (LISS) or treated with enzymes, and tested at 37°C, and

(c) the indirect antiglobulin test (p. 189), which is the most sensitive test for detecting IgG antibodies, must be used.

Potential problems in compatibility testing
1. *Incompatibility* can be demonstrated by one, several or all methods for one, several or all units of blood to be transfused. When incompatibility is found the following tests are carried out:
   a. the recipient's and the donor's blood groups are determined and in recipients with group A_2 or A_2B the presence of anti-A_1 is excluded;
   b. compatibility tests are repeated;
   c. the direct antiglobulin test, if not already completed, is carried·out;
   d. antibody screening is performed.
   A fresh sample of blood (at least 20 ml) may be required. Only units of blood which are compatible are issued for transfusion.

   When compatible blood is not available for transfusion to a patient with lifethreatening bleeding the consultant in charge of the patient may request, following discussion with the haematologist or a senior member of the blood bank staff, that the 'least incompatible' blood is issued for transfusion. When transfusing 'least incompatible' blood the procedure described on p. 90, 141 should be followed. It is essential to collect 20 to 40 ml of blood from the patient prior to transfusion with 'least incompatible' blood for further testing.
2. Following *massive transfusion* of ten or more units of blood virtually all the blood in the circulation is from the donors. Therefore modified and shortened compatibility tests, such as

the 'spin method', may be used instead of the standard procedure.

3. *Repeated transfusions* If the patient has been transfused more than 48 hours prior to compatibility testing, a fresh sample of blood must be provided, because a secondary (anamnestic) response of antibody production may begin in that time.

4. *Compatibility testing in a patient known to have auto- or alloantibodies* should be requested well in advance of the time set for transfusion because the search for compatible blood may last many hours, days or even weeks.

Issue of uncross-matched blood
In an emergency it may be necessary to transfuse the patient before the compatibility testing can be performed. Whenever the ABO and Rh(D) groups are known issue group specific blood. Group O blood is issued only when the ABO and Rh(D) groups are not known and the urgency does not allow for the blood grouping to be carried out. Group O Rh(D)-negative blood is issued for women and, if ample stocks are available, to men; men are, however, usually transfused with group O Rh(D)-positive blood.

The blood grouping and cross-matching procedures must always be started and completed. If blood is required before the procedures are completed, a short 'spin' technique is carried out and compatible blood issued at the request of the clinician in charge. If the completion of cross-matching reveals incompatibility of the unit of blood already issued, the ward or operating theatre should be immediately informed, the transfusion discontinued, the administration set changed and transfusion of compatible blood started as soon as it becomes available. The procedure described on p. 88 should be implemented.

The clinician requesting the release of uncross-matched blood is responsible for all the consequences of transfusion and he is required to sign an appropriate form before such blood can be issued.

Antibody screening and identification

Definition
Serological tests carried out on the patient's serum to detect the presence of an irregular antibody and identify its specificity.

Indications
Antibody screening is carried out in pregnant women, when investigating haemolytic disease of the newborn, haemolytic transfusion reaction or suspected immune haemolytic anaemia. It should be also performed in all prospective recipients of blood transfusion. All blood donors are screened for antibodies by transfusion centres.

Principle of antibody screening and identification
Antibody screening is carried out by testing the patient's serum against a panel of at least two types of red cells, each collected from a carefully selected group O donor. The panel should contain Rh(D)-positive and

Rh(D)-negative red cells. The procedures used for compatibility testing, including the antiglobulin test, are also used for antibody screening. When an antibody has been found in the patient's serum, it is fully identified by testing the patient's serum against a panel of red cells collected from six to 20 blood group O, fully phenotyped donors. The analysis of the pattern of agglutination provides identification of the antibody. The specificity of the antibody is confirmed by demonstrating the absence of the corresponding antigen on the patient's red cells (see below). The interpretation of results may be difficult if the patient has multiple antibodies or an antibody against a high frequency antigen. In patients with autoimmune haemolytic anaemia agglutination will occur with all red cells including the patient's own cells.

Potential problems in antibody identification are twofold:
1. the methods require high quality reagents as well as technical skill and experience, and erroneous results are not uncommon in inexperienced hands;
2. rare antibodies may elude identification for a long time. When either of the two problems is encountered help from a reference centre should be sought.

Red cell phenotype determination

Definition
Determination of the antigenic make-up of the patient's red cells by serological testing. This can be carried out for one antigen only or for one or several systems of antigens.

Indications
Red cell phenotyping is almost invariably carried out in conjunction with other tests used for investigating a patient with alloantibodies, neonates with haemolytic disease of the newborn and individuals participating in family studies for linkage investigation or paternity testing. It should also be done before starting long term transfusion regimes in patients with aplastic anaemia, pure red cell aplasia, thalassaemia major or sickle cell disease. Phenotyping for legal purposes and testing for paternity exclusion should be only carried out by pathologists licensed by the Home Office.

Principle of red cell phenotyping
The patient's red cells are tested with a selection of antisera each containing a specific antibody against one red cell antigen. The testing can be carried out for one antigen only, e.g. K, several antigens of one system, e.g. C, c, D, E and e in the Rhesus system, or for a large number of antigens, including the testing of saliva to establish the secretory status.

Potential problems in red cell phenotyping arise when old red cells or antisera are used and conflicting and inexplicable results are obtained. Also it may be difficult or indeed impossible to phenotype red cells coated with antibodies or drugs and red cells whose surface has been altered by the action of bacterial enzymes.

Antiglobulin test

Definition
A test used for demonstrating the presence of antibodies on the patient's red cells or in serum.

Indications
Used for investigating suspected immune haemolytic anaemia, a haemolytic transfusion reaction and haemolytic disease of the newborn and as a part of compatibility testing.

Principle of the antiglobulin test
Red cells coated with an incomplete antibody are easily agglutinated on incubation with antiglobulin serum. This is made by injecting an animal, usually a rabbit, with human serum, harvesting the immune serum and subsequently purifying it by absorption. A broad spectrum reagent or purified specific anti-IgG, anti-IgM, anti-IgA or anti-complement component (anti C_3d and anti-C_4) are available; they are used for determining the specificity of immunoglobulin or complement complex on red cells.

The direct antiglobulin test (DAT) is used for detecting the presence of antibodies on the red cells. Red cells coated with immunoglobulins agglutinate when antiglobulin serum is added.

The indirect antiglobulin test (IAT) is used for detecting the presence of an antibody in serum. First, 'control' red cells are incubated with the patient's serum to become coated with his antibody. The cells are washed and antiglobulin serum is then added; if antibody is attached to the cell surface agglutination will occur.

Interpretation of the results obtained by the DAT
A positive DAT indicates the presence of an antibody on the red cells. Further tests are required to establish its properties, e.g. its class (IgG, IgM, IgA or complement), subclass, complement binding capacity, etc. and its specificity. Occasionally, healthy persons have a positive DAT; the diagnosis of haemolysis therefore should not be based on the result of the DAT alone but there must also be evidence for haemolysis (hyperbilirubinaemia, haemoglobinaemia, reduced concentration of haptoglobin, increased urobilinogen in urine, haemoglobinuria, shortened ^{51}Cr red cells survival, reticulocytosis).

Tests for cold agglutinins

Definition
Tests aimed to detect the presence of and to quantify cold agglutinins in serum, to define their properties and to determine their specificity.

Indications

Investigation of patients with suspected haemolytic anaemia due to cold agglutinins (chronic cold haemagglutinin disease, lymphoma, infections, paroxysmal cold haemoglobinuria) and investigation of patients prior to cardio-pulmonary bypass or other procedures using hypothermia.

Principles of detection of cold agglutinins

Samples of venous blood must be collected using a syringe, needles and tubes warmed to 37°C. The sample of blood must be kept at 37°C while being transported to the laboratory and until the serum is separated from the cells.

1. *Presence* of cold agglutinins is demonstrated by incubation at 20°C and below.
2. *Specificity* of cold agglutinins is established using group O red cells from adults (for I antigen) and cord blood (for i antigen) and, when required, a panel of red cells (for P_1, M and other antigens), as well as enzyme treated cells to detect anti-Pr antibodies (see Table 14.1). The patient's own red cells are always used as a control.
3. *The thermal range* of cold agglutinins must be established. Only agglutinins which are reactive at 30°C or higher are clinically significant.

Interpretation

Cold agglutinins reactive at 4°C against either I, i and the patient's own cells or P_1, M or other antigens are not uncommon in the elderly. Antibodies with a titre higher than 1:128 and/or reactive at 30°C should be investigated further as they may be of clinical significance.

RECORD KEEPING

Blood banks should keep copies of (1) each request for blood group determination and compatibility testing, (2) the laboratory results, and (3) the report. In addition, the blood bank should keep a day book or sheet where all laboratory tests and observations are recorded, and a register for blood received, issued and returned to the transfusion centre. In the UK it is recommended that laboratory records are kept for at least one year. In view of the recommendation that patients' notes are kept for eight years after the last entry, it seems prudent to keep the record pertaining to transfusion of blood to patients for the same period of time. For children the notes are kept until they reach 25 years of age, and similarly blood transfusion records should be kept for the same period. In other countries the period of retention of all the records may be different and may be subject to legal requirements.

The report is usually presented on either the original request form or on its copy to avoid errors in transcribing the patient's identification. The report should contain all the results obtained and state the methods used.

When compatibility testing has been requested the report should state patient's blood group and list the identification numbers of units tested, their blood group and expiry date.

Patients' notes should contain reports of immunohaematological and of compatibility testing. Prior to transfusion of each unit of blood the unit identification number, blood group and expiry date and the result of compatibility testing must be checked by two members of the medical or nursing staff and recorded under signature.

Patients with antibodies usually have a permanent record in the blood bank. Their hospital notes are clearly marked either on the outside or inside the cover to indicate the presence and specificity of the antibody. The patients are also issued with a personal card stating the blood group and specificity of the antibody.

REFERENCES

BCSH Blood Group and Transfusion Task Force 1984 Guide lines on hospital blood bank documentation and procedures. The British Society for Haematology
Dacie A V, Lewis S M 1984 Practical haematology, 6th edn. Churchill Livingstone, Edinburgh
Hoffbrand A V, Lewis S M (eds) 1981 Postgraduate haematology, 2nd edn. Heinemann, London
Huestis D W, Bove J R, Busch S 1981 Practical blood transfusion. Little, Brown, Boston
Mollison P L 1983 Blood transfusion in clinical medicine, 7th edn. Blackwell Scientific, Oxford

APPENDIX I

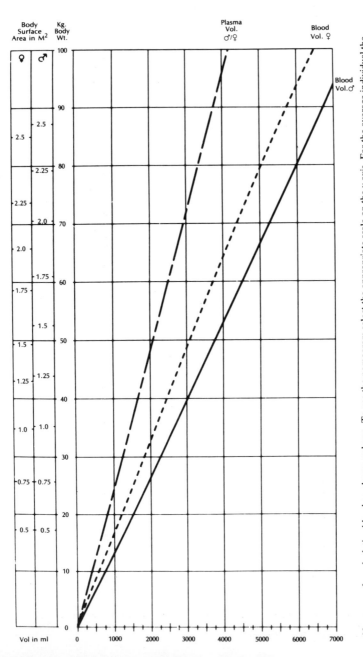

Nomogram for calculating blood or plasma volume. To use the nomogram select the appropriate scale on the y axis. For the average individual the scale in kg body weight should be used. In cases of excessive obesity or cachexia the body surface area, determined from the nomogram for calculating the body surface area of adults (Appendix II) should be used. Select the appropriate line for the value desired: plasma volume, or blood volume — for men or women, then draw the line from the intercept to the x axis to determine the correct volume. (Reproduced from *Blood component therapy. A physician's handbook*, 3rd edn, 1981, with kind permission of the American Association of Blood Banks)

APPENDIX II

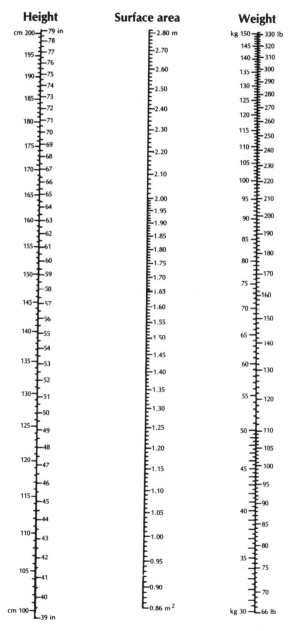

Height — **Surface area** — **Weight**

Height	Surface area	Weight
cm 200 — 79 in	2.80 m	kg 150 — 330 lb
— 78	2.70	145 — 320
195 — 77		140 — 310
— 76	2.60	135 — 300
190 — 75	2.50	130 — 290
— 74		125 — 280
185 — 73	2.40	120 — 270
— 72		— 260
180 — 71	2.30	115 — 250
— 70		110 — 240
175 — 69	2.20	105 — 230
— 68		100 — 220
170 — 67	2.10	
— 66		95 — 210
165 — 65	2.00	90 — 200
— 64	1.95 / 1.90	85 — 190
160 — 63	1.85	80 — 180
— 62	1.80	
155 — 61	1.75	75 — 170
— 60	1.70	
150 — 59	1.65	70 — 160
— 58	1.60	— 150
145 — 57	1.55	65 — 140
— 56	1.50	
140 — 55	1.45	60 — 130
— 54	1.40	
135 — 53	1.35	55 — 120
— 52	1.30	
130 — 51	1.25	50 — 110
— 50	1.20	— 105
125 — 49	1.15	45 — 100
— 48		— 95
120 — 47	1.10	40 — 90
— 46	1.05	— 85
115 — 45	1.00	— 80
— 44	0.95	35 — 75
110 — 43	0.90	— 70
— 42		
105 — 41		
— 40		
cm 100 — 39 in	0.86 m^2	kg 30 — 66 lb

Nomogram for calculating the body surface area of adults. (Reproduced from *Blood components therapy. A physician's handbook*, 3rd edn, 1981, with kind permission of the American Association of Blood Banks)

APPENDIX III

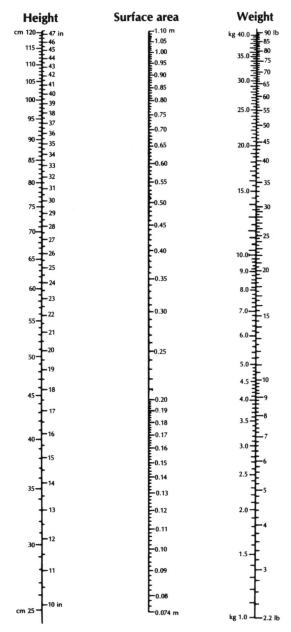

Height	Surface area	Weight

Nomogram for calculating the body surface area of children. (Reproduced from *Blood component therapy. A physician's handbook*, 3rd edn, 1981, with kind permission of the American Association of Blood Banks)

INDEX